C000261541

Dedication

I dedicate this book to my amazing mum.
Without all your hard work and sacrifices,
it would never have been possible.

Love and miss you.

Published by
www.elitepublishingacademy.com

All rights reserved.

No part of this book may be reproduced in any form by photocopying or
any electronic or mechanical means, including information storage or
retrieval systems, without permissions in writing from both the
copyright owner and the publisher of the book.

First Edition published 2017
© Phil Agostino

Printed and bound in Great Britain by
www.elitepublishingacademy.com

A catalogue record for this book
is available from The British Library
ISBN

978-1-910090-85-5

LOSE the FLAB FAST

The Quick, Dirty and UNCENSORED SECRETS to extraordinary fitness success without LIVING at the gym, DUMB-ARSE fad diets *or* Third World HUNGER

Phil Agostino

What Business Owners Are Saying About Lose The Flab Fast

"After more than twenty years working in an office I was suffering from a bad back, poor posture and a general lack of fitness. After getting some treatment for my back, I started a course of Pilates with Phil, but he soon suggested that to improve further I would benefit from spending time in the gym and especially using free weights to strengthen my core. I was slightly concerned as I had the idea that using free weights was the home of young "gym bunnies" and would not provide me with any aerobic fitness that I also wanted to improve. However, both of these concerns were put to bed quite quickly.

The main benefit of working with Phil is that everything is explained, demonstrated and reinforced so that it achieves the maximum potential. Only having time for two whole sessions per week means that I need to maximise the benefits from the gym. Whilst it takes time to learn the correct technique, it is well worth it, as I was able to increase the weights quickly and get a good hard aerobic exercise. Now watching some of the 'gym bunnies' with poor and ineffective technique, listening to Phil explain what I am doing right while I exercise, demonstrates that the time spent was well worth it.

I have been working with Phil for four years and the benefits are quite marked. I now stand upright and don't walk 'pigeon-toed' - saving a lot of money on shoe leather. My general fitness is much better as I now run up all stairs as a matter of course, and I can ski for hours in all terrains without hurting (the core strength helps posture, and hence technique, in so many sports from skiing to golf to cycling), and I have even been sun-bathing without a shirt on for the first time since I was a student. I generally feel better and with a busy job I feel that my mind is a lot sharper, as I am not tired so often.

The other strength of Phil is he understands fully the effect that diet has on lifestyle too. As I do not generally have a bad diet, since I don't eat cakes, snacks etc. nor drink alcohol too much, I find that my weight is fairly stable. However, having done one session of ten weeks when I lost a pound a week, I am about to embark on a second session to hopefully get that six-pack I have always desired. Having spent time in the gym, there are improvements to my chest, arms and legs etc., but to get that extra toning and leanness does need dedication to stick to a fairly strict diet. Phil's diet plan is easy to follow and if you use common sense you can also make it work for you - I have a fairly busy social life and I adapt my meals to accommodate when I am out for an evening or weekend. However, unlike the gym, the diet is about your motivation and cannot be influenced by Phil, apart from his encouragement.

Therefore, I feel that the time and money spent has been well worth it. Phil's attributes are that he is more mature and can speak to you effectively and efficiently. He is also someone who is personable so one-to-one time is enjoyable – as long as you do what he says!! He is good at pushing people and if you are happy to make it a partnership, it will work for you, too."

Paul Broom / Finance director

"I'm not one for reading books on fitness or health, despite having wanted to get fitter and lose weight for years. A lot of the time I thought I knew what to do, and figured the only stumbling block was my willpower and ability to stick to the rules.

Between family life and running my business, I'm pretty busy, and often use business as an excuse for having something unhealthy, but quick and easy.

This book, I found incredibly easy to read, despite my natural inclination to not really bother... maybe have a skim read but ultimately this is just another one of those "get slim fast" type books that do nothing but lighten your wallet.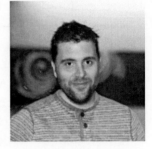

The thing is, Phil did two things with this book. First, he showed an immediate understanding of what it's like to be constantly battling with trying to get "the right diet". Getting to that breaking point and then thinking "screw it I'll start again later" and that later never comes until too much damage has been done. Second, he gives you everything you need to know in this book.

What stunned me, is that actually I had been going about

"dieting" all wrong for years. Looking to cut my calorie limit too low, and avoiding any "treat" like food or drink meaning I was quite simply, bored, dieting.

This book has allowed me to create an (easy) diet plan that let's me eat all the foods I want, but tracking it all in the right way so that I keep within my "limits" and keep on losing weight, week by week... and the beauty of this all is, I won't need to "stop dieting" once I reach my target weight, just make sure I'm doing the same thing (keeping to within the right limits) and for once, I'll keep it off.

If you're looking for a book that'll help you lose some weight, and you think nothing could possibly help you because of your crazy busy lifestyle, this is the book for you"

Ben Waters / Digital Magnet / www.digital-magnet.uk

"My main concern before working with Phil was whether I could transform my body without drugs, as a 40+ yo trainee, and whether I could do it injury free. I've had a lot of injuries over the years and injury prevention was critical. I also eat a whole food, plant based diet, and I'm well aware this is not a typical bodybuilder diet.

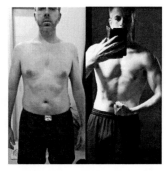

My worries quickly disappeared. Phil has been very supportive around the injury prevention issue and offered some good alternatives I'd not have considered on my own. The food was a non-issue and I've easily still to my plan even with on a non-conventional diet. The result is my body fat has reduced significantly, and I'm in better shape than I've been in years. I'll be able to carry that shape with me permanently now.

One of the things I liked most about working with Phil was the responsiveness. I needed a coach to be there in those moments I was weak, particularly around diet. I'm a very strong willed person, but put a big fucking cake in front of me and I'll destroy it. I needed Phil a couple of times through my program to help keep me off the shit food.

I would certainly recommend Phil's approaches to other people, because quite simply, it works."

Mark Cottle / Frontline

"When I look back at my 'before' picture I cannot believe the progress that I have made in just twelve weeks.

Phil's plans, advice and guidance helped me achieve my goal much sooner than I believed possible. For me the result has been transformational- not just in how I look but how I feel about myself.

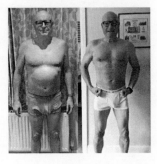

An unexpected but very welcome benefit has been a knock-on interest in health and fitness from my employees. This has resulted in measurable increases in productivity, energy and creativity. The net result has gone straight to the bottom line…amazing."

Tim Fitch / Invennt Ltd
www.invennt.com

"I was always one of those lucky people who could eat whatever he wanted and never put on an ounce of weight. Was. Because as soon as I hit 30, I started slowly piling on the pounds. Then two years ago, I started working for home. Suddenly I wasn't slowly piling on the pounds anymore — I was getting fat, fast.

One day I decided I had to do something about this... so I turned to YouTube. But what I found was a mess of confusing and contradictory advice. I bought some weights and played around with them... but I had no idea what I was doing and never really stuck with anything. Before I knew it, the weights were sitting in the bottom of my cupboard collecting dust. All the while my waist size was creeping up, and I felt like crap.

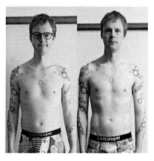

This is where Phil comes in. Someone I know worked with him and got impressive results. So I signed up.

The first thing Phil did was change my diet. He told me what to eat, and when. This was a bit of a revelation to me — I thought I was eating healthily already. Surely I didn't need to change my diet? It turned out that I definitely did. The next thing Phil did was create a bespoke training routine for me. The problem I'd had in the past trying to do things alone was that I had no idea what exercises I should do. Phil took the guesswork out of the whole thing.

I dropped around 6cm from my waist and 10cm from my stomach in just over two months, as well as added about 2cm to my arms (which I'm still working on, as well as improving my posture from years of sitting slumped over a computer).

I've got a lot more energy than I did just a few months ago, and just feel much better in general."

Julian Northbrook / Doing English
www.doingenglish.com

"As a doctor one thing that drives me nuts is when I read medical or fitness advice online or in print that is clearly wrong. Sadly you see this all the time – especially when it comes to health and fitness.

So when Phil asked me to review his book "Lose the flab fast!" I didn't know quite what to expect. I knew he was a competitive bodybuilder but had no idea how much he had "bought into" some of the useless fads that are out there.

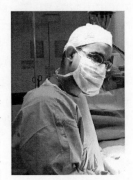

Having read his book I'm delighted to say that my fears were totally unfounded.

Because Phil is clearly an expert on exercise and nutrition. And in "Lose the flab fast!" he shows you step-by-step how to achieve your fitness and weight goals, all fully backed up by science and with none of the pretentious rubbish you read from some of the other "fitness gurus" out there.

So whether you're looking to lose the lard to look better on the beach and in the bedroom, or you've hit middle aged spread and want to get fit so you're around a while longer for your kids, "Lose the flab fast" is the book you need.

Put Phil's simple diet and exercise plan into action and you too can achieve the results his clients have without starving yourself or spending hours and hours each day in the gym."

Dr. Dev Lall
BSc(HONS)
MB ChB FRCS(Eng.)
FRCS(Gen.Surg.)
Surgeon
www.privatepracticeexpert.co.uk

"Several years back my scale stopped at 123 kgs. That was the turning point when the pain of being lardy got higher than doing something about it.

And doing something I did. I lost in excess of 40 kgs in just a few months.

All well and good.

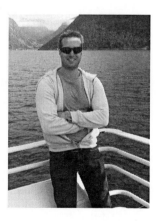

The problem was, I'd done it all wrong. In the process I'd not only lost flab, but precious muscle mass as well. And over the course of the next few years, I slowly gained weight again, until I once again was Mr. Lardy. Not as corpulent as before, for sure, and I'd trained hard and gained plenty of muscle mass as well, but still way too heavy.

I needed to lose weight again, but retain muscle mass.

Cue Phil Agostino.

See, Phil's a bodybuilder. As the hackneyed old saying

goes; he talks the talk and walks the walk. Woo woo and fairy tale free. What he gives you in his book and through his coaching programmes are simple and powerful principles and strategies to help you lose weight and retain your muscle mass - and help you stay there.

If you're new to Phil, reading the book will introduce you to his world - a world where simplicity rules. Not overly complicated and confusing diets that are impossible to stick to.

Sure, nothing comes without a price. You'd have to do the work, which means doing what Phil says. To the letter.

But if you do, you'll discover that his promise in the book title actually holds true. You too, like me and his other clients, can actually lose the flab fast without living at the gym, dumb-arse fad diets or third world hunger."

Vegard Svanberg

The Breakfast that changed my life.

I had heard of Phil Agostino from a business colleague of mine who had mentioned him several times via his newsletter how he had improved his health and physique by utilising Phil's methods and techniques. Jon was already into fitness, so I thought that Phil was more for people who were already getting some good results and knew their way around the gym - It turns out; I was flat out wrong about that assumption.

It was not until I met with another acquaintance who had invited me to join him for breakfast in London, UK who also had become a client of Phil's that my eyes were opened. Tim explained to me during that breakfast about the success he had personally had in losing weight and regaining a 32" waist by directly working with Phil.

Now I've struggled with my weight for as long as I can remember. I was a very fat teenager, and in my 20's I did manage to lose much of that weight. Over the past 30 odd years or so, it all came back, and it's been tough going.

Believe you me, I have tried many a diet and while short term they may have worked I always ended up regaining the weight (and then some) back.

I made a mental decision right after that breakfast that I would contact Phil as soon as I got back to Canada and start a program with him.

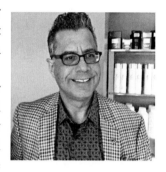

Have been working with Phil for about the past three months and getting some positive results. My whole attitude towards health and exercise has changed 100% for the better.

After having read Phil's book, I can tell you that he backs up all his recommendations with science and research. That was quite important to me. I am tired of reading books on diet and fitness that are full of half-baked theories and carry very little substance or quasi-scientific research usually skewed in the author's favour.

Unfortunately, there are many out there. You won't find any of that nonsense in Phil's book.

Ray Khan / Toronto, Canada

Lose the Flab Fast

The Quick, Dirty, and Uncensored Secrets to Extraordinary Fitness Success Without Living At The Gym, Dumb-Arse Fad Diets or Third World Hunger

Phil Agostino

Table of Contents

Foreword

About eight years ago I was a little porker: 44 years old, 190lb, and only 5'5" tall, with a waistline of 39 ½ inches. And far too little of it was muscle.

In other words I was fat.

But not only was I fat, but I was miserable with it.

See, I knew I was fat but the thought of doing anything about it left me feeling even worse than being fat did, because I knew a fair bit about diet and exercise and the whole grinding process stretched ahead of me like an unclimbable peak.

But I wasn't disgusted enough to do too much about it – I was still drinking my bottle of wine most nights and making excuses not to do anything about it. You know, eating the pizza and the chips, and convincing myself it didn't matter too much.

And then something remarkable happened... I saw an article on the BBC website about a guy who was quite a few older than I was, and had been vastly overweight. Warned by the doc he was going to drop dead pretty much any day, he'd lost some ridiculous amount of weight (fourteen stones or something equally bonkers), mostly by cycling. And just reading that article made me realise, suddenly, the pain of where I was hurt a lot more than the pain of doing something about it.

So, I took my old bike out that same day, got a half mile up the road, and thought I was going to die (which, disgusted me even more as I thought I was quite fit). I changed my diet, started lifting the weights, and persevered. And within a very short period of time I was down to 11 stone, working out three times a week, and able to cycle pretty much indefinitely, with the only constraint being on my time.

Success story, eh?

Not quite.

Because being human… I let things slide. I never got anywhere near as fat as I was before, but my weight did bounce around between 11 and 12 stones, and no matter how hard I tried, I could never attain that mean, lean, muscular look you see on all the male models (Me? Vain? Too fucking right). And this carried on for a few years — never getting too out of shape, but never hitting that elusive goal, either.

And then in June 2016, after a particularly heavy night out in London with some mates, I realised if I was ever going to get the look I wanted I was going to have to get some expert help. Man, I was 51, and figured if I couldn't do it with a PT, then it was never going to happen at all.

No pressure, then.

Around that time I'd been swapping messages with Phil on Facebook — mostly filthy and inappropriate jokes. I liked the guy personally and got on with him, and from his photos and the stuff he posted I could see he knew his stuff. So I asked him about working with him, we had a quick chat over Skype, and I decided to take the plunge.

We started on July 4th, 2016, and I made one rule for

myself right at the start: unless it was clearly ridiculous or physically impossible for me (because of my age I have the usual collection of creaks, cracks, crunches, grinds, aches, pains and injuries a lifetime tends to confer upon us), whatever he said to do I'd do.

And that's what I did.

And the results?

Spectacular.

You can see the pictures for yourself (and they're not Photoshopped), but in short they were phenomenal. For the first couple of weeks nothing happened as I got used to my new workouts and Phil got my calories right, but then... oh, my. The fat just melted off me. I sent in underwear-shots weekly — front, side, and back — and the changes were visible from one week to the next. And within just 5 months I'd gone from a squishy little old bloke to a ripped and muscular 9% body fat.

Best of all?

None of it was complicated, none of it was especially hard, and until the last week or so, the dieting wasn't in the least challenging (the weekly Skiploads or "face stuffing" helped there).

Now just bear in mind:

- I was 51yo. Not old, but not a youngster, either.

- I don't have insanely good genetics. I've never been obese, especially not as a kid, and that helps. So does "muscle memory" from the times when I've been more muscular than I was at the beginning of that summer. But otherwise, I'm just an average Joe when it comes to genetics. Very few people are fat because of genetics or their metabolisms: they're fat because they eat too much and exercise too little.

- It wasn't difficult. While I wouldn't say it was easy, it was simple and didn't required a massive change in how I lived. I wasn't buried in the gym for hours at a time, and I was doing the same amount of cycling and shit I was doing before. Nor did I find the dieting particularly hard.

- Phil was easily able to tailor my workouts around me, personally, and my working style so it didn't interrupt my working day and how I ran my business (a vital secret to any weight-loss is it has to be convenient and easy).

- I had a niggling back injury that severely curtailed my iron-pumping for about a month. Some days I could barely walk, and even lifting the weights onto the bars for the exercises I could do was a challenge.

- I had my business mastermind week and a trip to London in that time. True, I did restrict my food and alcohol intake to much less than it would normally be at those times, but I fell off the wagon somewhat, and over the days I was there I wasn't able to exercise at all. What I achieved in 5 months I could have done in 3½ without injury or interruption.

- While I lost comparatively little weight, my body composition changed dramatically. In other words, I lost loads of fat and put on loads of muscle. At 51. While in calorie-deficit. That's nuts.

Question is... why was it so important for me to get lean and shit? After all, I was fit and healthy, and I wasn't even that fat, not compared with most people.

The answer was pretty simple: I didn't want to look just "OK" naked; I wanted to look amazing.

I also never want to be the "Fat Dad" my kids are embarrassed by (that alone is a huge motivator for me).

Call it vanity if you like, but it's nice to get admiring looks from women (and daggers of hatred and envy from men, especially those who are decades younger), simply because you look good. And while I'm not obsessive about any of this stuff, I do take it seriously because it's a serious business. I'm not chasing my youth, but I am chasing health and vitality.

Why?

Because when you look good and you're physically fit, you feel good, all the way through. And when you feel good you're simply a lot more effective and productive... plus it's pretty cool being chased down the road by hot Eastern European chicks from the local supermarket, throwing their knickers at you (no, really, that actually happens to me on a regular basis).

But it goes way beyond my health and personal life.

Because it's helped my business immeasurably, too.

Look, science tells us regular workouts form what's called a "gateway habit". The necessary disciplines bleed out into other areas of your life and everything improves. I first noticed this after my Fat Jon Moment, and when I was moved to take action, it all became a lot easier (now exercise is a deeply ingrained habit in my life, to the point where it's not uncomfortable not to do it).

And the discipline required to do this (which is surprisingly easy to maintain because the goals were suddenly so important to me) permeated every part of my life and business, and I've not looked back since.

Now, I did all this working closely with Phil... and I knew not everyone is in a position to do that. He's busy, he's exclusive, and he's very expensive (and rightly so).

So that's why I urged him — to the point of bullying — to write this book.

And in your hands you are now holding the definitive guide to fat loss and body-recomposition for the busy business owner or executive. Everything you need to effect a massive transformation in your body quickly and easily without massive disruption to your life and business is within these pages. It's easy to understand and — most important of all — easy to do.

So a simple tip if you want to grow your business — get fit, healthy, and lean.

You'll have more energy, more discipline, and you'll just feel better about yourself and everything else in the world.

And the best way to do it?

Read this book and do what I did — whatever Phil says.

Jon McCulloch, The Evil Bald Genius
www.evilbaldgenius.com

Preface

Congratulations... and welcome to my world. By buying this book, you are already moving in the right direction towards improving your health, your fitness and to losing that bit of that flab that has accumulated over many months, or possibly years. Choosing to read this book should prove to be a great decision for your wellbeing and even your business, provided you take the action needed, of course. If you're struggling with weight gain, energy issues, or you are just generally fed up with feeling like shit, then hold on tight, because over the course of the next 200 or so pages, you'll have the answers that you seek. This will have a huge impact on how you look at exercise, dieting, and your understanding of how these things can fit alongside a life full of business meetings, travelling, stress and, well... life in general, really.

I'm Phil Agostino, and I help entrepreneurs and business owners Lose The Flab FAST without them needing to live at the gym, and eat cold chicken from a plastic container. Well, not unless they want to. By the time you have got through the pages in this book you will have all the tools you need to finally get this problem solved.

Obviously, all I can do is steer you in the right direction by providing you with what I believe are the best ways to lose weight and get fit, as well as my experience in doing so for hundreds of clients, over the past 12 years. I can't do the work for you. And that is exactly what you are going to have to do if you are to get the most from this book. It's going to take plenty of hard work, commitment, and some sacrifices to Lose The Flab FAST.

Now, you've probably heard a lot of that before, but the reason why I know what you've heard or read in the past was wrong for you is simple: you still needed my book. Therefore, you still have the same problems to solve. Problems that I am more than confident that I can help you solve.

Why so confident? Well, I've been doing this for a long time – well over a decade now – and I have coached many guys just like you, who spend a lot of time travelling for business, who eat out a large percentage of the time, who often rely on hotel gyms and restaurants, and who have the pressure of having to be "sociable" with new and existing clients, without wanting to come across as "weird". Yeah, those things are a pain in the butt, and it would be far easier if you had a nine-to-five in the office and never went anywhere else, of course, but that doesn't mean it cannot be done. I've proven (well, my clients have) that it can be done, and I'm going to teach you how.

My clients are not stupid. Many of them run multi-million-pound businesses, and so they definitely won't invest in someone who they don't trust to help them, especially given the prices that I charge them. You can rest assured that when it comes to fitness, health, and losing that beer belly your wife now mocks you for, that I know exactly what I'm doing. This will become more apparent as you delve deeper into this book.

Finally, please go into this book with an open mind. Many guys come to me already having their own ideas and beliefs on the "best" way to lose weight, and sometimes changing these views can be difficult. Ironic, really, when by coming to me, they are acknowledging that they don't know what the hell they're doing.

To add some weight (pun intended) to my credentials, here is a photo of me from 2015, when I did my first body-building competition:

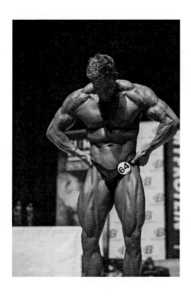

Chapter 1

Lose the Flab Fast

There are so many reasons why I decided to write this book, the main one being that I want you to be able to go away and Lose The Flab FAST, in a way that's simple, effective and, if you actually do what I suggest, life-changing.

I've been doing this a long time now, and quite frankly, I'm shocked that I still get asked the same questions and see the same mistakes being made that I did back when I started. This is one of the reasons I decided to write this book. With the Internet, and the government having become more and more focused on stopping the UK's ever-growing waistline from getting any worse, you would assume that finding the information needed to help you lose a few pounds would be fairly straightforward. Obviously, this isn't the case at all! In fact, Public Health England (PHE) recently stated that a staggering 77% of men aged 40-60 (i.e. most of you reading this right now) are classed as overweight or obese (Gov.uk, 2017).

That, my friends, is as depressing to me as it is unsurprising. It's unsurprising because I see it every day. Running a busy online fitness consulting business allows me to witness the same excuses, problems and frustrations that stops guys like you from getting into the shape you'd love to be in. I get to evaluate plenty of food diaries (awful), training plans (embarrassing), and, of course, answer a lot of questions on a day to day basis. I also have plenty of successful entrepreneurs and business owners on my Facebook and on my email list, and this allows me to witness how poor their lifestyles really are. Whether it's endless photos of high calorie meals in restaurants or simply just photos of them looking like crap, it's obvious that even though many of you are brilliant at taking care of business, you suck at taking care of yourselves.

Recently this type of body – soft, squishy and lacking any real muscle – has infamously been called the "dad bod"[1] . I disagree though; it isn't being a dad that's made guys like you look this way. Hell, some of you might not even have kids. The real reason you look this way is because building and running a successful business has become more of a priority than looking after yourself. That is the reason why I refer to a body like this as the "business bod". The business bod is the result of guys just like you – eating on the go, entertaining clients in restaurants, being away from home week after week, long days, sleepless nights, and hoping your daily caffeine habit will see you through to the end of the day, where you will most likely eat whatever is simple and easy, i.e. junk foods and take-aways.

Everything I experience just further highlights how badly most guys want to burn some flab, build a little muscle, have enough energy to stay motivated to run their business, and still want to bang their wives at the end of the day. Surely,

---

1   For those who haven't seen this floating around the media, then the dad bod is basically a slang term for describing the bodies of middle-aged men, usually with kids. Although you certainly don't need to be a dad to have a body like this.

this isn't too much to ask. Well, it will be, if you keep listening to the rubbish many fitness professions, and fitness magazines are spewing out of their arses on a daily basis.

It's not totally your fault, though. Going back to what I said about having the internet earlier, let's be honest: not all the information on there is really that good. Unfortunately, anyone can write a blog, upload a YouTube video, and worst of all... advertise themselves as a "personal trainer" online. Unlike when I started, you can become a fully "qualified" personal trainer (in the UK, at least) in just six weeks; so you can see exactly why the information out there for you guys to consume can, at times, be very poor. Anyway, I think I've made my point.

Truth be told, I've made plenty of the same mistakes as you, and annoyingly, just like most of you, I also wasn't born with great genetics. I'm 5ft 6 tall, and even after a couple of years of fairly consistent training I was still only about 60kg (9.5st). I had legs smaller than some of the girls I worked with, and my arms were a joke. Now, usually the silver-lining to being the skinny kid is that you have a six-pack. Sadly, I didn't even have that! I tend to get fat easily, too. I remember coming home one summer from university, and walking through the door, to be greeted by my mum with "God, you've got really fat". In fact, this is how I still looked in my early 20's, with a few years of training under my belt:

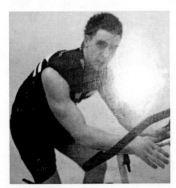

This is from my first ever personal trainer 'bio' board. I must have been 21, possibly 22. Take note of how skinny I was, for someone training 5 times a week, for several years.

12

See...small arms, small legs, and had you asked me to "lift my top", that would most certainly have been a "no" as well. It's safe to say that I know what it's like to hate how I look, feel self-conscious about how my clothes fit me, and the pain and frustration that comes with all that. However, it's okay, because I learnt that with the right advice, and a lot of hard work and consistency, I could mould myself into something that I'm happy with, as well as help others to do the same.

There you have it. I felt that there needed to be a book that specifically catered for busy, successful, middle-aged entrepreneurs and business owners, that wasn't full of the usual bullshit, doesn't perpetuate the nonsense that most fitness magazines often publish, and, above all else, is simple and easy to understand. Oh, and it goes without saying that it would get you guys some actual results along the way. The same kind of results I'm known for getting my 1-2-1 clients.

I'm not going to go "full science" on you in this book, as I want it to be as easy to read, understand and implement as possible; however, I've found that most of the guys I work with (being highly intelligent) are often interested in knowing why I'm suggesting certain things. Therefore, don't expect it to be totally dumbed down. Honestly, I also believe this is an important part of the process. People tend to respect and follow information more when it's backed up by science and reason. Along with a little science, there will be plenty of anecdotes about former clients and myself. Whilst on the subject of "former clients", I'll add that although this book is written with men in mind, that I will use stories and examples that involve past female clients, as I guarantee that you will still learn something from their experiences.

Even as a trainer and coach myself, I've made my fair share of mistakes, whether with myself or with clients in the early days. As you can imagine, I've got the good, the bad and the ugly to talk about, and I feel relating the science to my real-world experiences will serve to cement the importance of what I am teaching you. Additionally, just for good measure, there will most likely be a few swear words and a rather blunt, to the point attitude from me. This is just me being me. I don't like to sugarcoat things. As a coach, it doesn't serve me well to be afraid to tell my clients what they need to hear (nor does it serve them well). It's only right I'm the same in this book. If there are sections that are uncomfortable to read, then you know that we are on the right track.

With all that being said, I feel we should dive right in. By the end of this book, you will understand nutrition, be able create your own diet and training plan (one that actually works), and know how to get the most from the gym. You will also be armed to deal with things you may not have considered, such as peer pressure and dealing with crappy friends and family.

"Where should I actually begin?"

In the following sections of the book, I'm going to cover some things I consider to be very important, even if they don't directly relate to the structure of your training or your diet. Saying "I want to lose some weight" is one thing, but what precedes you actually getting started may be the difference between success and failure. I encourage you guys to take a step back and understand what I'm talking about in these sections first.

In the following chapters, we shall discuss how to correctly determine your goals, and no, "Lose my beer belly" isn't good enough, believe me. We'll also look at some other aspects that you will most likely not have even considered, but that I feel will make your new lifestyle changes happen a lot smoother – so long as you apply them. Don't be lazy. The stuff covered here, in my opinion, is just as important as the training and diet plan you use.

Goal setting – "Err, I just wanna lose some weight"

To keep this book well rounded and ensure it's as practical as possible, I wanted to start at the very beginning, in the same way that I would if you contacted me for some 1-2-1 coaching. One of the first things we would discuss can be summed up in the following two questions:

1. What do you want to achieve?
2. Why do you want to achieve it?

I know what most guys will say when I ask them what their goals are. I can't begin to estimate how many times I've asked that question over the years to hear something along the lines of "I just want to get fit and tone up, really", or "I want to feel better and have more energy". That really isn't a fucking goal. It's akin to me asking you, "What do you want to achieve with your business this year?" and you replying, "I want to grow it". No shit. So even before we look at how to create a great diet and training programme and ban the missus from buying your favourite take-aways, let's take a step back and think about what it is you really want to achieve.

Are Your Goals "SMART"

A good goal(s) will follow the "SMART" principle, ideally. That is, your goals should be:

- Specific
- Measurable
- Attainable

- Relevant and rewarding to you
- Time-bound

Right, so let's break these down and discuss them in a little more detail.

Specific

This one should be pretty obvious, but as I've said above, most of you will have goals that are the complete opposite of specific, and are vague at best. What you want are goals that are well defined and, if possible, quantifiable. For example, instead of "I want to lose weight and feel better", you might say:

1. I want to lose 10kg.
2. I would like to fit into 32" waist trousers.
3. I would like to be able to perform 20 full push-ups.
4. I don't want to suffer from back and neck pain anymore.

If a client has goals that are mainly visual, but isn't all that clear on what it would look like to them or find it difficult to describe, then I'll often have them find me a photograph of someone who has the kind of body they would like – just so that it's clear to them what it is they are actually aiming to accomplish.

As a coach, this helps me greatly, and you too will find that having specific, clear goals will give you a better sense of direction. Oftentimes, I'll prompt a client to really think about it by asking them, "In a year from now, if you've achieved your goal, how will you feel? How will it improve your life, and your business?" This usually encourages them to really consider what it is they are looking to achieve, and more importantly, what it would feel like to finally get there.

For many of you, it will be to wake up in the morning feeling like you have more energy, so that you feel motivated and inspired to keep working hard on your business, while still having the energy to spend time with your families. Like many of my clients, you might enjoy sports such as golf, skiing and cycling, and want to be able to do these without pain, soreness and a concern for your health. Many of you will have the goal of being able to enjoy your favourite sports and hobbies, regardless of your age.

Spend some quality time looking at what it is you want to achieve on a deeper level and make your goals as specific as possible.

Measurable

There are plenty of ways that goals that involve fat loss and muscle building can be measured and tracked, all of which will be discussed in greater detail later in this book. These include:

- Fasted body weight,
- Body measurements,
- Caliper testing[2]

Be sure to track these from the start. You'd be surprised how many men come to me having no idea of any of these, even though they may have already begun trying to achieve their goals.

You can also look for other things to measure that aren't related to how you look, for example:

---

2   Caliper testing is where skin folds are measured using special calipers at certain points on the body, usually in areas that hold more fat. These measurements can then be used to estimate someone's body fat percentage, if required.

- What is your energy on a scale of 1-10?
- How much pain are injuries and niggles giving you on a scale of 1-10?
- Are performances improving, i.e. are you able to complete a 5km faster?

There are so many things you can measure to ensure you keep track of your progress; but be sure that your goal has several components that can be measured and tracked.

Attainable

Having goals that you're capable of achieving is very important and I can't stress this enough. Now, that doesn't mean you should "set the bar" too low. There is something to be said for being ambitious. I'm sure there aren't many professional footballers or Olympic medalists who didn't dream of making it to that level from the very beginning. That being said, most of you reading this book will be 40+, have businesses to run, children to look after, a wife at home nagging you, past injuries and so on. Let's be frank; you're probably not going to look like Arnold Schwarzenegger or Lou Ferrigno[3] anytime soon, or set any world records.

That doesn't mean that you're unable to make some drastic changes to your fitness, health and your body. You can. Just be realistic about what you want to achieve and ensure you consider this in relation to how much time, energy and dedication you're willing to invest into it. Remember that, like most things, the more you put in, the more you'll get out. Those of you reading this who are willing to (and who can) sacrifice plenty of time for your training and cardio, can stick to the plan consistently, and learn to "miss out" on foods

---

3   Lou Ferrigno, if you didn't already know, is the guy who first played The Hulk, in The Incredible Hulk TV series.

and drinks you enjoy from time to time, will achieve more than those of you who aren't. What you can achieve will ultimately be down to how much you are willing to work for it – much like you would have done to get your business up and running, and to ensure it remains successful.

Why is this so important? One reason is motivation. If you're chasing almost impossible goals, it will be very difficult to stay focused on diet and training, because it will "blind" you from appreciating the progress that you are making. Losing 3kg in a few weeks is motivating; yet losing the same 3kg isn't as motivating if you were expecting to lose 8kg. The last thing you want is to lose motivation and begin to tell yourself you're "failing" simply because you aimed too high.

Secondly, aiming too high and never achieving what you want will often lead to disappointment and frustration, and in the end, you'll say "Fuck this" and give up. Going back to Arnold, he was my hero growing up. I still remember my dad and I watching the documentary Pumping Iron for the first time, and wanting to have a body just like his. I would have done anything to look like him, and over the years I would say that I pretty much have – yet I still look nothing like him. I'm nowhere near the level of a pro bodybuilder. Luckily, I'm older and much wiser now, and so I understand that in the same way as some people are just better at math, or art, there are those that will make the kind of progress in the gym that I couldn't make in an eternity. It's very easy to become envious of other people's bodies, even for guys, and it can only work to your detriment if you end up doing so. I should know, because I've been there.

Don't set yourself up for disappointment before you've even begun. Please don't let that put you off having goals that are going to be difficult though. Difficult and unattainable are totally different. The key is to understand the difference and find the right goals.

For weight loss goals, the recommended weekly loss is usually 0.5-1% of your current body weight. This means that if you're 90kg, you could safely lose 0.4 and 0.9kg per week (1-2lbs roughly speaking). Bear in mind people will often lose 2-3 times that in the first week or two, and this is due to water weight being lost. After that initial period, you should expect the weight drops to be a lot more modest.

Relevant to you

Your goals have to be yours, and yours alone. Now, you might be thinking "Well, whose goals could they be but mine?". This might come as a surprise, but they will often actually be somebody else's. It can be fairly common if you've been in a relationship long enough, and have come to the point where you've become much more honest than you used to be.

Let me give an example. Me and my girlfriend are both very competitive, have high expectations of ourselves and have been together long enough to not really "hold back" all that much. I'm also her coach, so believe me, if I think her butt is getting too fat, then you know full well I'm going to tell her. (I enjoy it as well, but let's keep that to ourselves.) This really isn't that uncommon. I was chatting to a new client recently and one of the things he mentioned was that his wife had started to make comments about his "beer belly" and how he had "let himself go". Women like a dig, don't they? I'm sure more than a handful of you reading this have experienced this at some point. During my slightly "fatter" phase while I was trying to gain some muscle, my girlfriend took a lot of delight in telling me I had "moobs[4]".

---

4   For those unfamiliar with 'moobs', it is a colloquialism for 'man-boobs'. Creative, right?

In fact, having some moobs might even be one of the reasons why you're actually reading my book.

Many of you will listen to this "heartless bullying" (because that's what it is, right?) and will decide to do something about it. This isn't a bad thing, obviously, but sometimes this will force guys into making the decision to change their lifestyles before they've actually thought about whether or not they are ready to do so.

If you're purely doing it to please someone else and not for yourself, then I really think you increase your chances of failure. It's like those children who choose their career path based on what their parents want them to do, knowing full well they're passionate about something completely different. Trying to please their parents is not often going to be enough of a reason for them to want to work hard, and chances are they'll end up miserable or will quit. This can happen with health and fitness goals as well.

Get your head in the game first. Sit down and find a goal you truly believe in, and that inspires you. Your chances of success will greatly improve by doing so.

Time-bound

This one speaks to me on a personal level and may do to you as well. I don't know many people that can get things done in a timely fashion without some sort of deadline. As the deadline creeps up on you, the pressure increases, and this will often give people a nice kick up the arse.

Without a clear end date set for you to achieve your goal, you'll more than likely put it off. It's definitely easier if you have something to keep you accountable, like a wedding, a holiday, or a business event in the diary that you want to look and feel your best for. If you're just doing this for yourself then you'll need to be strict with yourself. Set an end date and put a lot of energy into sticking to that deadline. With no real pressure, it's easy to find yourself thinking "Ah, a few days off won't hurt", because you know that you can "move the goal posts" without any real repercussions.

As discussed above, the recommended weight loss per week is 0.5-1% of your current body weight. If we stick with the 90kg example, then at 0.5-0.9kg you could have the goal of losing 3kg-5.4kg over the first 6 weeks. Bear in mind that you might gain some muscle or hold water on the diet that will affect your actual weight loss, which means that we can take those figures with a pinch of salt; but the point is we have a clear goal to achieve in a certain timeframe, which means you can keep yourself accountable with weekly check-ins and ensure you stay on track. This 100% beats the usual, vague "I want to lose weight" sentiment with no more detail than that. You could do the same with more performance based goals as well. For example, you could aim to be able to run a certain number of miles by week six, or be able to cover a certain distance in a certain amount of time. Again, the value of this is to keep you focused and on track.

I will add that it's usually better to give yourself a little more time than you actually need. Even with all the planning in the world, life does tend to want to kick us in the balls from time to time. Aim for a good balance between having enough time to get the job done, and enough pressure to keep you focused on it.

Setting multiple goals for continued focus, accountability and progress

Goals can and should be broken up into even smaller goals that help lead you to your final goal. Therefore, instead of concentrating on the final "end prize" – which can often feel "a million miles away" and equally as difficult – you will concentrate on smaller milestones along the way. You often will find that those "mini wins" along the way keep you motivated to stay on track.

Your **long-term goal** is, of course, the final desired outcome. Of course, long-term goals will change over time, but everyone will have something they want to achieve in that moment in time. For physique enhancement goals, then, "long-term" will often be 12-16 weeks. That is enough time for most guys who are hard-working and committed to radically change their bodies, their health, and feel like a different person. This also represents the longest I would ever really have someone diet for, before taking some time off. I'll talk about that more in another chapter.

But it doesn't hurt to think of goals that are even farther into the future than that. For example, in my first competition, I competed at 71kg in the under 80kg class. It therefore makes sense to have a long-term goal of several years, with the aim of one day competing around 78-80kg. To be honest I don't overly concentrate on that goal because it's too far away, but in the back of my mind, this is what all of my other goals are working towards. It's no different to maybe having the goal of selling your company at a certain point. You know it isn't close, but it keeps you moving in the right direction. Having a big (albeit realistic) goal is nice, provided you're aware that it will sometimes take years to achieve. For me, I'm fine with that, and if you are too, it doesn't hurt to have something to aim for.

Your **medium-term goal** will usually be something you aim to achieve around the halfway point. For example, if you are aiming to lose 10kg in 12 weeks, by week 5 you should have lost around 5kg. This again purely allows you to assess whether or not you are on track; and if not, changes can be made to your plan. There can be other medium-term goals too, such as ensuring that after a certain amount of time, you're regularly training with intensity and confidence. Often, what I'll do is assess what a client is "weakest" at doing well. For many, it will be sticking to their food plans consistently.

What I'll often do is give them targets to achieve along the way. For example, if they struggle with eating out for most meals, I would ask them to prepare at least 50% of their meals at home, thus reducing the need to eat out. As adherence to their plan improves over time, I might then ask them to prepare more of their own meals per week. Another example could be that they are missing morning gym sessions because they're too tired to wake up early enough. Over the first several weeks, a medium-term goal might be to ensure they consistently make it to the gym 3 mornings a week, from maybe 1. Get creative with these goals and use them to analyse where you seem to let yourself down, and use these shorter-term targets to stay in control and to keep ensuring you're making progress.

Short-term goals are often made up of several mini goals. These could literally be hour to hour, day to day, week to week, or training session to training session. Those who find it difficult to stay on track will often find that having these mini checkpoints along the way stop them going off the rails. A short-term goal that I currently have is to aim to be in bed, regularly, by 11pm. For years, I went to bed at closer to 1am and then got up at around 5.30am. I've recently found that with the extra training I'm doing, and with business being very busy, that wasn't quite enough sleep to recover sufficiently. The thing is, I like staying up later, so I literally need that 11pm bedtime target to keep me on track, as I know that when I stick to it, my training performance increases and I work much better.

One area that I demand clients really commit to is tracking their training sessions. In every training session, the exercises, weights and reps performed should be recorded so that they have something to beat at their next session. For example, if you can do five press-ups in week one of your training, then the following week you would aim for 6-10 reps. It's this tracking that will, over time, ensure that you get stronger in the gym, and this will lead to a better physique, less fat and more strength.

Short-term weight goals are also extremely important so that you are made to be accountable for your progress. Ultimately, the reason for short-term weekly goals is to ensure you're going to make the end goal in time; and if not, at least you can analyse why you might not, and can look for solutions to any problems you have and then make the relevant changes to your plan.

Interestingly, I've found over the years that the guys who begin to actually enjoy their training often do better long-term than those who just view it as an inconvenience and a necessary evil. You have to consider that eventually you'll lose the weight you wanted to lose, that holiday will have come and gone, and you will feel lot better – what now? At this point, without the initial goals that inspired you to begin in the first place, maintaining your new lifestyle will be very difficult. There is a good chance that you will stop and return to your old lifestyle, therefore quickly regressing back to where you started i.e. fat and unhealthy. If you can get to the point where you begin to view making progress in the gym as a goal in itself, carrying on becomes a lot easier.

My current client Paul came to me with a shoulder injury, a bad back and a little bit of a belly at the age of 47. His background was running and he therefore had no experience with using a gym or weight training. Once I'd fixed his injuries, we moved onto the weights, and now, 4 years later, he's not only inspired by looking and feeling better and being able to ski better than he could 20 years ago, but he takes great delight in being able to progressively add more weight to the bar, week by week. This has definitely been something that's kept him motivated to continue his training all these years with me. Had he only been motivated by improving his goal of fixing his shoulder injury, there's a good chance he would have stopped working with me long ago, he wouldn't have gained the leg and core strength to improve his skiing, and he certainly wouldn't have learnt how to maintain his weight, even with of all his work and social commitments. It's actually very nice to see a guy go from weak and injured to someone who, at 51, goes into the gym with the energy, determination and the ambition of someone half his age.

The 5 Whys: "So WHY do you actually want to lose weight?"

Several years ago, I was diagnosed with Ulcerative colitis, an inflammatory bowel disease that resulted in me losing something crazy like 3 stone (19kg) in around two weeks. Not only that, but the dodgy bowels and diarrhoea that came with it made it impossible for me to even leave the house. Seriously, I literally had seconds between thinking "I need the toilet" and "Bollocks, too late". I was sitting on the toilet as often as 100 times a day! Being a single guy in my late twenties, who still enjoyed nights out, loved bodybuilding, and made his living standing in front of crowds of people teaching fitness classes, this was a dilemma, to say the least. Even worse was that I got to the point where none of my medications were working and it was beginning to look like I might need surgery and a colostomy bag.

There was no way in hell I was going to let this happen, and after some extensive research I found a book that provided a diet that had helped a lot of people in my situation. The drawback was that foods like pizza, cake and chocolate weren't on the list of "legal" foods. Bugger. Regardless, I followed that diet to the letter for 13 months. For over a year I didn't touch anything that wasn't "legal". I had the willpower of a monk in a strip club! My symptoms cleared up so well that I was able to stop ALL of my medication, I regained my weight and strength, and no longer had to worry about crapping my pants every time the toilet was out of sight.

The question I'm often asked, and this will lead me to the point of this entire section, is how I managed to stay so committed to such a restrictive diet for so long. The answer is very simple, I assure you. Regaining my health, getting my life back and avoiding surgery simply far outweighed my desire to eat the foods I was craving. I just placed more value on my health than being able to eat certain foods, something that most people are embarrassingly poor at doing. The real key to my commitment was that I had a very good reason, or "why", for following the diet – and that is what this section is about. It's an important one as it may be the very thing that stops you from halfheartedly trying to achieve your goals and ensures you begin this 100% committed.

The "5 Whys" is something you may have heard of or even used in your business training. Wikipedia describes it like so:

"5 Whys is an iterative interrogative technique used to explore the cause-and-effect relationships underlying a particular problem. The primary goal of the technique is to determine the root cause of a defect or problem by repeating the question "Why?" (En.wikipedia.org, 2017).

In other words, you can use the 5 Whys as a way to dig deeper and find the real reason you want to achieve your goal(s). It encourages you to think carefully and then provide a unique, personal and emotional reason behind wanting it.

The ultimate reason to do this is so that you place some value on your goal, and isn't just something arbitrary. Consider the perceived difference in value of a goal between a guy who thinks he "just wants to lose weight" compared to that same guy admitting he wants to lose weight because he can no longer play with his children and the guilt of this keeps him awake at night. The latter is a way more powerful motivator. This is why I found the diet needed to help my Colitis fairly easy to follow. The value of success was very high and very motivating.

So how do you do this yourself?

Very simply. You define your long-term goal, and then ask yourself why you really want to achieve that. You then ask why again, digging deeper and deeper until the real pain you're trying to get away from is revealed.

It might look something like this if I'm consulting with a new client:

> **Me:** "So what do you want to achieve while working with me, Dave?"

> **Dave:** "Well, I'd just like to lose a bit of weight and feel better."

> **Me:** "Okay, so why do you want to lose the weight. What is making you want to do that? What do mean by 'feel better?'"

> **Dave:** "I just feel a bit fat right now and I have very little energy in the mornings."

Me: "Ok, that's good. You're lacking energy. Why would having more energy help you? How will it improve things?"

Dave: "I'm tired all the time. I used to wake up full of life and be looking forward to doing some business. Now I wake up feeling like I've got a hangover. My mind is foggy and it takes me several alarms to get up. Once I am up, all

I think about is getting back to bed. It's affecting my productivity at work. If I'm honest, I also don't have much desire to sleep with my wife anymore. I get home, eat the wrong foods, and just go to sleep. This is definitely causing a strain on our marriage. I'm just too exhausted after a 15-hour day, you know?"

Me: "Okay, I get that a lot. Losing weight and getting fit will improve your business as you'll be more motivated and clear minded, while at the same mean you're able to maintain a better relationship with your wife. THERE is your 'why' that you must remind yourself of when you feel that the plan is too hard and you're considering stopping. Can you see the value of this and how achieving those goals are more important than the odd beer or take-away, mate?"

Dave: "Definitely, Phil! That is a much better way to look at my goals! It really puts things into perspective."

This should be rather uncomfortable to do for many of you, and quite rightly so. In the example above, which is fairly common, "Dave" has not only admitted to struggling with his business, but also that it's putting a strain on his relationship with his wife. This is something that many men will experience, especially as they get older and more successful. The point is, and I'll be blunt here, sometimes you will need a very good fucking reason to get your arse in the gym, stop yourself from binge eating after a long day at work, and maybe even say "no" to the odd beer with your mates, to achieve something great. You won't do those things if you merely want to "lose weight".

You just have to get to that point where, in your mind, you know why you want to change and are happy to acknowledge and accept it. Not easy, I assure you, but well worth it. I'll be frank now: if knowing you'll be around to see your kids grow up, having many more years with your wife, and being able to earn more money in your business aren't good enough reasons to get your shit together, then you really need to look at your priorities. Sadly, this is the case for many. I once had a client start with me, and one of their reasons for wanting to lose weight was that they felt "guilty" for not having the energy to play with their kids. Still, that particular person only lasted about eight weeks. Shocking. Discover your "why" at the very beginning and give yourself a much better chance of success.

Do this NOW:

1. Write out 2-4 goals that you want to achieve in the next 12-16 weeks that are specific, measurable, attainable, are realistic and have a time-scale.

2. For each of your goals use the 5 Whys exercise to get a better understanding of what is really behind those goals. Find your "pain". The thing that is going to drive you forward no matter what.

Chapter 2

How to make dieting a "piece of cake"

Let's tackle the subject of dieting, something that's clearly the most difficult part of the weight loss equation to stick to. I'm not surprised. To get great results, in most cases, you will only be required to exercise for roughly 3-10 hours a week (a mere 1.8-6% of your time), whereas you must be accountable to your diet anytime you are not asleep. A much greater commitment, I'm sure you'll agree. It's therefore usually far easier to slip up with the diet, especially if you don't know how the hell you're meant to be going about it correctly. That's not to say you will definitely find getting to the gym easy; but in my experience, it's definitely the part most people get into the habit of faster. The question, then, is this: how do you stick to your nutrition plan well enough to make sure all the training you're doing is worthwhile? Well, that's what this section aims to help you with.

I will guarantee that a large percentage of you reading this will have attempted to lose weight already at some point in time. For some of you, this might be something you've battled with over and over for much of your lives.

The statistics on weight gain, dieting and people's ability

to maintain any weight they have lost are sadly pretty poor. I can state rather confidently, though, that the reason most of you have been unsuccessful is because you will have done everything you possibly could have to make your diet more difficult than it needed to be. Fortunately, this book that you have in your hand right now will prove to solve this problem.

The purpose of this entire chapter is for me to explain, and therefore ensure, that dieting is simple and easy to implement into your busy lives. Making it more sustainable, long-term, than any other way of dieting you've ever tried in the past. Sure, you probably all know that you need to eat less (and/or move more) to lose weight, and most of you will have a fairly good idea of what healthy eating should be like, yet this still isn't enough information for most people to get the results they want. What I find are the real issues though is that most guys will follow dumb-arse fad diets that are too strict, highly restrictive, lead to excessive hunger, and have a ton of weird rules to follow, making them a terrible choice. In the following sections, I'm going to ensure you completely understand exactly how you should go about structuring your nutrition plan, for a lifetime of success.

Calorie requirements - "How many calories should I eat each day?"

The fundamental part of weight loss

If we consider a hierarchy of what aspects of nutrition are the most important for successful weight loss, at the very top would be the need to create a daily calorie deficit. In other words, your body must use more energy (through metabolism, exercise, activity and a load of other things) than the energy you provide your body (through the food and drink you consume) every day. Essentially, it's this energy balance that dictates whether you will gain, lose or maintain your weight.

To keep this simple, let's imagine that your body requires 2000 calories per day to maintain your weight. 2000 calories is enough to do everything that you're required to do, from being able to function, go to work, walk, chase the kids, etc. If you provide your body with 2000 calories, then you have energy balance and your weight will not change. However, if you create a negative energy balance, through either consuming a little less food and drink, moving a little more or a combination of both, then your weight will go down. So, for example if you begin to eat 1500 calories each day, instead of your usual 2000, then you have created a daily calorie deficit of 500 calories. Over the course of the week this would equate to a total calorie deficit of 3500 calories[5], and that would give you roughly 0.5kg of weight loss.

Now please, please, please remember this! In the same way that's it's fundamental that your businesses turnover exceeds your expenditure in order to be profitable, it is fundamental that you're consistently in a calorie deficit if you want to lose weight. Do not let anyone tell you any differently. There are many "scientists" and "coaches" who still, regardless of all the science, believe that the energy balance isn't important and like to put the blame on things like sugar being responsible for people gaining weight. Remember this throughout the book and when you go to plan your own diet plan (which you will do after reading this).

It seems simple so far, right? You'd think so, but it isn't. Many people, even when studied for research, will underestimate the number of calories they consume each day. It's also something I've witnessed myself over the years with the food diaries I've evaluated for clients. It is very easily

---

5   500 (calories) x 7 (days) = 3500 weekly calorie deficit.

done if you are not mindful of your food choices, portion sizes, and all the things that you consume, then conveniently forget about. You know, like that biscuit you had at a friend's house, the milk you added to your teas and coffees, and the oil you threw into the pan to cook with. They all have calories, and those calories all affect the calorie deficit you are trying to maintain throughout the week. This is why, later on in this book, we will discuss how you can easily track your daily calorie intake to ensure you're totally accountable to it, and are able to easily make adjustments, if you are not getting the results you desire.

The thing most will get wrong

Now, we know that a large percentage of people are consuming way more calories than they require each day. We know this because so many of them are overweight, and they continue to gain more and more weight. Funnily though, when someone starts a diet it's very common that they will go from far too many calories straight to far too few calories, in an attempt to lose weight as fast as possible. Several years ago, I had a girl come to work with me whose diet, under the advice of her current personal trainer, contained only 800-1000 calories per day, even though she was training for a marathon and weightlifting. The result? Her body was weak, lacked muscle, was holding body fat around her midsection (the area where she stores her most stubborn body fat), had an underactive thyroid, and she had lost her menstrual cycle. Hardly ideal, wouldn't you agree?

In order to fix that situation, I had to increase her calories for some time, while essentially "fattening" her up. It took about a year before we were able to begin dieting again. The second time was, of course, much different and obviously successful. Why am I telling you this? Well, this actually happens a lot. I would say that maybe 50% of the people who come to work with me have fallen into the trap of trying to overdo it with copious amounts of exercise along with a very low-calorie diet. Those clients, like the client I was just talking about, all have one thing in common: they aren't able to effectively lose any body fat. We always have to spend several weeks, to months, correcting the damage done. They come to me to diet, and get told they can't. But this is always the best course of action, and in the long run taking a step back always proves worthwhile. I'm telling you this because, just as eating too much food will stop you losing weight, going to the opposite end of the spectrum will also cause lots of issues.

Recommended weekly weight loss

The key then, is to aim to lose a healthy, sustainable amount of weight each week of around 0.5-1% of your current body weight per week.

> *Example: If you weigh 90 kg, then a weekly loss of 0.5 and 0.9 kg would be recommended*

Truth be told, most people can safely get away with and sustain a weekly loss of 0.5-1.0kg, especially in the beginning. Just bear in mind that as your body fat levels get lower, and you have been dieting longer, you will usually have to accept that the drops you experience will become smaller. Just so you know, to lose that amount per week, you would need to be in a daily calorie deficit of 500-1000 calories for an entire week.

Calculating your daily caloric needs

So that you can avoid the issues associated with lowering

your calories too much in the beginning, I recommend you use this equation to find a good "start point" for your plan:

> *Body weight (kg) x 22-26 = Estimated calorie requirement per day*
> *Example: 90 kg man would do 90kg x 22-26 = 1980-2340*

Obviously, when you use the equation above, you will have to determine whether to start at the high end or the low end of the spectrum. As you can see from the example, two guys weighing 90kg may require a difference in calories of several hundred. It would be nice if I could be a little more "black and white"; however, I can't, because this sort of thing is highly individual.

What I would then suggest you do is base your start point on your current situation. If you are fairly active, have a job where you move a lot, or are already doing some training, then it makes sense that you will need more calories than if you hardly move at all. At the end of the day, starting your calories on the higher end of the spectrum, even if you do not need them, will never be a bad thing. At worst, you will just not make progress in that first week, but you will know that you simply need to lower your calorie intake in week 2. That's hardly an issue. In fact, I'd prefer this option over the alternative, where you underestimate your calorie requirements, lose too much weight in the first week and then have to consider adding calories back in. For most of my clients, I will start them off slightly higher for this very reason.

There are other ways to do these calculations and if you do a quick search online for "basal metabolic rate calculators[6]",

6 Your basal metabolic rate (BMR) is the number of calories your body would require to function if you simply rested all day. From here, most calculators will then add on extra calories based on your activity level to give you a more accurate recommendation.

you'll find several online calculators that will allow you to input more information, like your height, age and activity level. The thing is, when all is said and done, most of the time those more complex calculators will give a calorie requirement very close to the method I've provided you with. Plus, keep in mind that these calculations are always just a start point. I can't stress this enough. Your job is to follow your estimated recommended calorie requirements for several days and evaluate what results you get. Based on how the first 7-10 days go, you can simply adjust your daily calories, up or down, in order to improve the results you're getting (more on that in a later chapter).

Of course, you may well get a nearly perfect week, and in those cases I want you to remember the old saying: "If it ain't broke, don't fix it" – it's no different from something that is working very well in your business. Ride it out and get the most from it; just be sure to monitor it and have a plan ready for when it does eventually begin to produce poorer results. Until then, enjoy the progress, and relax.

Calorie budgeting "I've got a business lunch this week. What do I do?"

Something that's very important to understand is that you do not have to eat the same number of calories each day, in a linear fashion. This doesn't allow for much flexibility within your diet for things like weddings, business meetings and family dinners, where you might want to enjoy yourself without ruining all your hard work. Well, that can be done. Instead of using your daily calorie requirements, you can calculate what your weekly calorie requirements are. Those calories can then be distributed in a non-linear fashion to provide some extra calories on the days you might need them. Traditionally, in bodybuilding this is done so that more calories are provided on the days that you train, in order to provide more fuel and to improve recovery. This leaves fewer calories for your rest days when, in reality, you don't really require them.

Let's use a 90kg man as an example:

Assume our 90kg man (who trains 3x a week) needs ~2000 calories each day to lose 0.5kg over a week. Over the course of the week his TOTAL calorie requirements are ~14,000. Instead of eating 2000 calories each day he could split his calories like this:

Monday (gym training) = 2200 calories
Tuesday (rest day) = 1850 calories
Wednesday (gym training) = 2200 calories
Thursday (rest day) = 1850 calories
Friday (rest day) = 1850 calories
Saturday (gym training) = 2200 calories
Sunday (rest day) = 1850 calories

The total is still 14,000 over the week and so he would still lose 0.5kg.

This principle can also be used for social events. Let's imagine the same 90kg guy had an important business event on a Thursday night. He could split his calories like this:

Monday = 1650 calories
Tuesday = 1650 calories
Wednesday = 1650 calories
Thursday (business event) = 4000 calories
Friday = 1650 calories
Saturday = 1650 calories
Sunday = 1650 calories

The total is still ~14000 (13,900 to be precise), yet he has more calories "in the bank" for that day to use for a dessert or a glass of wine. Again, his weight loss by the end would still be 0.5kg, the same as if he just evenly distributed each day with the same number of calories. Cool, right? This is a very effective strategy I use with my clients that have more social and business commitments.

Some caveats:

1. Regardless of how low your calories are, you must maintain your protein where it's meant to be.
2. This isn't used as a way of creating a starve/binge cycle. I don't suggest you have days of NO food just to be a fat pig at the weekend.
3. I still want clients to make sensible choices. Having some calories in the bank is NOT the same as it being a day off the diet completely. Stick to meat and veg for the main. Don't have 10 glasses of wine, etc – do enough to enjoy yourself and not feel weird.

Something to consider

That pretty much sums up the subject of calories, but I want to add something very important to this before moving on. It's highly likely that if you eat the calories recommended from the formula above, it will be more food than you are used to, especially once you begin choosing foods that are more filling. In fact, I would estimate that 80-85% of new clients will complain that they can't eat all their food in the first few weeks. Ironic, considering that they often come to me complaining of always being starving! But it highlights that many guys, especially those with busy schedules, will be used to undereating (and then binging on easy to eat foods in the evening) and therefore will find their new plan a little bit of a shock to the system. Don't freak out. You won't suddenly gain a shit load of weight, believe me.

In most cases, after a few weeks, your metabolism will improve (read: that's important) and you'll soon find that amount of food way more tolerable. You may even begin to experience some hunger at this point. Not a bad thing, within reason. Not to mention you will most likely have fewer cravings and have more energy day to day and for exercise. With that being said, I need you to go into this new project with an open mind and be ready to try something new.

Macronutrients: "Macros? What the hell are they?"

You now know how many calories you need to consume each day, so that's step 1 ticked off. For many of you, that will be something you have never actually calculated, but I hope you can now see why that is vitally important to this whole book. It's not really an exaggeration to say that without that last section on calories, everything else we cover will be suboptimal.

For step 2, we are going to look at how and why you must break your daily calorie intake into certain amounts of macronutrients. Macronutrients are simply the protein, fats, and carbohydrates you have in your diet.

If calories are the king, then macros are the queen

I remember doing a fat loss diet many years ago after I'd finished uni to correct that final year of sleepless nights, excessive alcohol and (genuinely) living on pizza. I looked a mess. For that diet, I focused solely on my daily calorie intake. This was a mistake, and one that fortunately you won't have to make. Although I lost weight on the scale, that weight was clearly not all good weight, i.e. I definitely lost some muscle as well. You've seen the photo of me back then, and I certainly didn't have much muscle to lose. The last thing you want to do after slogging away lifting weights and sticking to a regimented diet is to lose muscle!

My issue was that by focussing on my calorie intake only, I was not taking into consideration where those calories were coming from, i.e. how much protein, fats and carbs I was getting from my food. Looking back, I can easily say that I was relying so heavily on carbs that I wasn't getting enough protein or fats for me to maintain muscle and have optimal health. Following a diet like this will drastically affect how you look at the end of your diet. Your goal is maximum fat loss, with minimal muscle loss. Ideally, you will at the very least maintain your muscle mass, and for those who are new to lifting weights, or returning to training after a long layoff, it isn't uncommon to actually gain new (or regain old) muscle.

During that diet, I massively under-ate protein, maybe having half of what I needed through a shake or two and some chicken. I didn't get any essential fats, because I didn't add olive oil to meals, I don't particularly like nuts and avocados, and I wasn't supplementing with fish oils. Therefore, my diet was probably ~70% carbohydrates, and to be honest, a lot of those carbs were consumed through poorer eating choices (such as cereals and chocolate) because I was teaching a lot of fitness classes (3-4 hours per day!) and told myself that I needed them for the energy. Something else I've learnt over the years is that most people don't need as many calories or carbs as they believe they do. Especially those for sit at a desk for 8-10 hours a day, drive to and from work, and then spend their evenings sat watching the tv. You're worlds apart from the calorie (and carb) requirements of someone like a builder. This is certainly something to consider when you calculate your energy requirements for the day.

Don't get me wrong, I'm certainly not saying that high carb diets don't work for fat loss, they very much do, but having high carbs at the expense of a good percentage of protein and fats will not be optimal. Remember that although your energy balance is the most important part of fat loss, thinking about where you get those calories from certainly has some value also. Thinking back to that hierarchy of fat loss we discussed earlier, your macronutrient ratio comes in as a solid 2nd after calorie intake, as you will learn in greater detail in this section.

I'm going to go through how you can determine how many grams of protein, fats and carbs you need per day to lose body fat, feel great and ensure you maintain (and sometimes even build) as much muscle as possible.

Something to understand is that unless you're doing this completely wrong, like I explained I had done above, then you can be pretty flexible with your macro breakdown. The most common myth, for example, is that you must eat a low carb diet to lose weight. Nearly everyone I speak to who has just begun a diet will say something along the lines of "I've completely cut out bread" (because we all know that bread is the devil, right?), but what they fail to understand is that when enough protein is being eaten, low carb diets don't outperform high(er) carb diets for fat loss (Naude et al., 2014).

Now, having said that, certain macro breakdowns will make one person feel great and another one feel lousy. A good example is the ketogenic diet, popularised by Dr. Atkins, which some people absolutely love! Yet you give someone else next to no carbs and they will feel awful, even after the initial period where the body is becoming accustomed to the new diet. Personally, I am not a fan of high carb diets, because I love carbs. Yes, you read that right! I will tend to choose to have my carbs on the lower end of the spectrum, having enough to maintain my training intensity, because I tend to want to overeat carbs. Dieting is hard enough as it is, and I don't want to spend every waking hour thinking about my next carb hit. Give me one chocolate bar to eat and I'll want to eat 20. Limit my carbs a little and I can train well, feel full, and almost completely eradicate my cravings. This is, for me, is the best I can feel on a diet.

What am I saying? Well, there is no perfect diet, I'm afraid. The "perfect" diet is the one you can stick to long enough to get some fucking results and not spend all day, every day, bitching and whining that you're craving, hungry and pissed off. The key, then, is to do some trial and error. Therefore, the calculations I give you on how to work out your macro needs will have ranges, and it's your job to play around with your diet and see where within those parameters you need to be. Protein is going to be pretty much set the same for everyone (relative to body weight of course), and there is a certain amount of essential fats you will want to ensure you adhere to, but the carbs can vary quite a bit.

Protein – "I'm struggling to eat all the protein!"

Protein is made up of amino acids and is the building block of all the tissues and cells in the entire body. Therefore, adequate protein intake from our diet is essential for optimal growth, repair and the building of new muscle.

In this section, I'm going to discuss several reasons for why you should prioritise protein in your diet, especially while trying to lose weight.

Before we get onto the benefits of higher protein levels and my recommendations, I am going to address several common health concerns that I hear from clients. The last thing I want is you to do is ignore this vital section of the book because your wife's, Pilates instructors, cousins, doctor, said that eating a high protein will kill you. It will not. So here are common health concerns associated with high protein (often from meat consumption).

Kidney damage

Although high protein diets are usually not recommended for people who already have some kidney damage, there doesn't seem to be the need for this precaution if you have healthy kidneys (Martin, Armstrong and Rodriguez, 2005). One study looked at the potential health risks of high protein diets in athletes and bodybuilders, consuming 2.8g of protein per kilo of bodyweight (considered high) and concluded that protein levels up to this amount had no ill effects on their kidneys (Poortmans and Dellalieux, 2000). Therefore, unless you have an existing kidney problem, a little extra protein isn't going to hurt. If you do have concerns, though, I would recommend speaking with your GP. Personally, I've been eating as much as 3.4kg of protein per kilo of body weight for years with no problems. Wonderful, steak all round then!

Cancer (particularly colon) and heart disease.

This is something that gets brought up on a regular basis, and some association has been shown between high protein intake from red meat and increases in health issues such as cancer and heart disease. For example, researchers at the Harvard School of Public Health observed data from two studies that included 121,342 men and women, who had no cardiovascular disease or cancer initially. Following these peoples diets for more than 20 years they found that eating one 85g serving of unprocessed red meat (beef, pork, or lamb) each day caused a 13% increased risk of death. That figure rose to 20% for consuming one serving of processed red meats such as bacon, hot dogs, sausage, salami and bologna (Sun, 2012).

Now, the problem is that these studies are done in large populations and usually just look at that one single factor: the fact that those people ate red meat as part of their diets. Those studies, being epidemiological, mean that the bigger picture isn't being considered. They can't take into consideration other lifestyle factors that affect your health. Remember that health is multifactorial! Those people who tend to frequently eat fatty red meats are often overweight, consume unhealthy amounts of alcohol, smoke, don't exercise, and the rest of their diet is shit. All of these factors play a huge role in the overall health equation. Is it really any surprise that they had an increased risk of death?

Now consider someone like myself. I eat one serving of red meat every day. I tend to choose a cut lower in fat, however, often opting for anything that's 5% fat or less. From time to time, I'll eat something higher in fat, like lamb, because it's my favourite meat. I exercise several times a week, I watch the rest of my diet, ensure I consume veggies and fruits, and I'm far from overweight. I probably drink one, maybe two small ciders a MONTH, and I've never smoked. All my blood tests show that I'm in good health. In short, my overall lifestyle is pretty spot on, 90% of the time. My risk of cancer and heart disease is therefore also significantly lower because of this, even though I do eat red meat every day.

Things get very blurred when you simply start to pigeonhole all meats into being "unhealthy", as well. There is a huge health difference between a fresh cut of steak with the fat trimmed off and some highly processed, ready cooked pepperoni, for example. Especially given that meats that aren't processed don't increase inflammation nor do they increase your risk of heart disease (Micha, Michas and Mozaffarian,

2012). Something to consider if someone suggests that a diet high in meat and protein can cause heart disease.

As M. Hill concludes in the paper 'Meat, cancer and dietary advice to the public' (Hill, 2002):

> *"Far from being supportive, the epidemiological data does not justify this claim. A large mass of evidence is presented from case-control studies and prospective studies, in which the data from Europe are not consistent with those from the United States. This is because of the different contexts (in terms of meal composition) within which meat is consumed in different countries. In fact, the epidemiological data are much more consistent with there being a protective role for fruit, vegetables and whole grain cereals and no role for meat in colorectal cancer, and a protective role in gastric cancer."*

Bottom line: High protein diets are fine, even when the protein is coming from red meats. I suggest you choose low fat varieties, like 4% fat beef mince, more often than not. Also ensure that you eat an adequate amount of fruit, whole-grain cereals and veggies, because they have been shown to protect people from disease.

With that out of the way, here are the reasons why you should ensure you prioritise the amount of quality protein you consume in your diet. This is essential, and why I believe it's the most important macro to get right.

Protein will help burn calories

The "thermic effect of food", or "TEF", is the amount that your metabolic rate increases (above normal rates) after eating a meal, due to the food within that meal needing to be processed and digested. In other words, when you eat, a certain percentage of the calories you've consumed are actually burned off and therefore can't impact your weight. Protein has the highest TEF at around 20-30% of the calories you consume being "used" to digest the food. Compare this to carbs with a TEF of just 5-10% and fat with a fairly useless 0-3% (Acheson, 1993).

To put that into perspective, let's imagine you consumed 200 calories from protein, fats and carbs (on their own), the TEF would account for the following loss of calories:

- Protein = 40-60 calories
- Carbs = 10-20 calories
- Fats = 0-6 calories

You can see why having a diet higher in protein may be of use when it comes to helping create a negative energy balance. It also proves to be another excellent reason to consider where your calories come from, and not just how many you consume. This is something I've already discussed, of course.

Obviously, we rarely eat protein, fat or carbs in isolation, and so these numbers will vary when you eat a meal with a mixture of all three. That said, increasing the protein will increase the TEF of a particular meal (Westerterp, 2004). I will say that in the grand scheme of things, this effect on your metabolism is rather small; however, every little bit helps, so it would be silly to not to consider it as part of your overall plan.

The feeling of fullness

At some point in a diet, a time will come when the meals you consume no longer fill you up as much as they used to. This is because of a hormone called Leptin. Leptin is produced by fat cells, and one of its roles is to tell your body how much fat you have and how much food you're eating. Its job really is to help you regulate your energy balance by controlling what you eat.

As you lose body fat, Leptin levels drop. This tells the brain you are not eating, and sure enough, your body, being too smart for its own good, tries to encourage you to correct this. From an evolutionary point of view, the Leptin is trying to prevent you from starving to death. It does this by stopping you from feeling full after you eat. A person who never feels full up following a meal (and also feels hungry) will, of course, have a bigger chance of binging once their willpower says, "No more". This is an easy way to ruin your diet.

When I dieted for my competition, I'd wait for two to three hours for my meal, eat my child-sized portion in like two minutes, and then instantly start feeling hungry and sick again. It was awful! You can blame evolution for this. It hasn't realised that there is plenty of food to go around (in some places at least), and that, in fact, you're not starving yourself, but just attempting to correct the effects of being a gluttonous pig in order to feel better, live longer and look the best you can.

I've digressed a little there, but knowing what I've just explained will help you understand why the protein in your meals is important, and that reason is: protein is more filling than fats and carbs (Astrup, 2005). This is why a large proportion of new clients I work with will initially find that they're unable to eat all of their daily calories. They are usually not accustomed to eating that amount of protein on a daily basis. In my experience, the majority of the time, when I assess a new client's food diary, the most obvious thing letting them down will be the lack of protein they're eating.

In the real world, the practical implication of this is fundamental to success: increased adherence. Many of you will choose to diet in a way that leaves you overly hungry. This will inevitably become extremely difficult to follow for a period of time that will yield results. With all other variables being equal, the diet that keeps you feeling fullest will usually be the easiest for most to follow, and this increases your chances of success. Therefore, I recommend that you make the protein in your meals a priority before other macros, especially the carbs.

Maintaining muscle

You may get sick of me mentioning muscle throughout this book, and that's fine, as long as by the time you've finished reading it, you can see why I've made such a meal of it (pun intended).

For a lot of you, your goals will not only be to shed some flab, but to build some muscle, as well, especially in areas like your arms, chest and shoulders. That's great! What you have to remember is that when you're dieting to lose weight, you can lose it from muscle, fat, or a combination of both. Clearly, it's not going to be ideal to lose 10kg of body weight if half of it is muscle. No shit, right?

I'm 100% certain that none of you want to end up "skinny", frail, and feeling weaker than a kitten. Therefore, it's vital that you make maintaining (or even building) some muscle a priority. During a diet, because you're training, doing aerobic work and trying to stay active, all whilst in a calorie deficit (and often eating less carbs), your body may, at times, have to use protein as a fuel source. Can you guess where it will pinch that protein from if you're not careful? Yep, your hard-earned muscle! Nightmare! The problem is, even if you're providing your body with some protein through food, once it's used as fuel, there still needs to be enough left for its primary role – growth and repair. If your protein has been too low, your muscles won't get enough to be able to recover and grow from your training. This certainly isn't optimal. You'll counter this by providing your body with an optimal amount of protein throughout the day.

Recommended protein intake

We have now discussed the benefits of choosing a diet higher in protein, and I'm fairly confident I've compellingly argued my point. All we need to do now is discuss exactly how much you should eat each day.

Research on protein intake tends to vary, and will of course depend on the individual. You will not need as much protein if you aren't doing intense resistance training. I'm going to base these protein recommendations on the assumption that you will be doing some resistance training. The International Society of Sports Nutrition (ISSN) recommends that the protein needs for those exercising should be 1.4-2.0g per kg of bodyweight. Those doing resistance training, aiming to get stronger should aim for 1.6-2.0g per kilo of bodyweight (Campbell et al., 2007). There was also a recent review of studies on protein intake for lean athletes who are used to resistance training and restricting calories concluded that they needed 2.3g-3.1g of protein per kilo of bodyweight (Helms et al., 2014). So what we have is a spectrum to choose from starting at 1.6g per kg of bodyweight and ending at 3.1g per kilo of bodyweight.

Personally, for the reasons I've already stated above about the benefits of protein, and from what I've been taught by my mentor, I've always favoured the higher end of the spectrum for clients. I tend to start people at around 2.8g per kilo of bodyweight, and most do well at that start point.

```
┌─────────────────────────────────────┐
│  Protein Requirements:              │
│  1.6 - 3.1 per kg of bodyweight     │
└─────────────────────────────────────┘
```

```
┌─────────────────────────────────────┐
│  Example (90kg man):                │
│  1.6-3.1 x 90 = 144g - 279g per day │
│  (Of course, this would be rounded up/down to │
│  keep the maths easy, so let's call it 145-280g │
│  per day)                           │
└─────────────────────────────────────┘
```

I will add that those recommendations by Helms et al. were calculated for someone's lean body mass, which is your body weight without the fat. However, like I stated above, I've been using similar recommendations for years, even for total body weight, and so I feel you will be fine using that equation without having to have someone calculate (or worse, you trying to estimate) your lean body mass.

The question you might be asking yourself is, how do you know how high or low to go? If you're the 90kg guy I used in the example, then you of course could choose your daily intake to be 145g, 280g or somewhere in between. Well, in reality, there is no right or wrong answer, and so I suggest you choose it based on your preference. I will add that if you are very overweight, and therefore very heavy but with little muscle mass, then you'll be fine using the lower end of the scale.

Some of you will find it really hard to eat a diet high in protein, whereas some of you will love it. Find the best amount for yourself within the range you've calculated and you really can't go wrong. The main thing to consider is that the more protein you eat, the fewer calories you'll have left to use for fats and carbs. There is a delicate balance needed to ensure you get enough of each, and you will find this out simply with some trial and error until you find what works best for you and your lifestyle.

One final piece of information that is worth noting is that for every gram of protein you consume, you will get 4 calories – so 50g of protein will equate to 200 calories. Over the course of this chapter, you'll learn how many calories carbs and fats have per gram. This information is also relevant, which you will see shortly.

Dietary fat – "Won't eating fat make me fat?"

Ever since I can remember, diets low in fat have been promoted and recommended as being the healthiest and the best diets for weight loss. This started in the late 70's early 80's with dietary fat guidelines coming into the UK in 1983. These guidelines have now been shown to have been recommended "in the absence of supporting evidence" (Harcombe et al., 2016). Reducing fat intake became common advice for losing weight most likely because fat is so calorie dense. Fat provides us with 9 calories per gram, more than double protein and carbs, and so removing fat removes a lot of calories. As we have discussed numerous times now, it's your energy balance that determines weight loss. I'm sure this is becoming very clear, so I'll move on.

Even though fat, particularly saturated fat, isn't bad for you if your intake isn't excessive (Chowdhury et al., 2014, Siri-Tarino et al., 2015), the trend to put people off consuming fats has certainly left its mark. You only have to look on shop shelves, or watch a few adverts on TV, and you'll still see all the low-fat foods being promoted, although this has certainly reduced a lot over the past several years. I will mention here that trans fats have been shown to affect our health negatively, so all recommendations in this chapter will not actually include them.

Let's briefly look at the different types of fat. I'm sure you are aware of them:

1. Saturated fats
2. Polyunsaturated fats (omega 3 & 6)
3. Monounsaturated fats
4. Trans fats

(In a later chapter, I will compile a simple list of foods you can consume to get the right fats.)

Dietary fat intake is important for your health, having benefits such as decreasing inflammation, improving hormone levels, absorbing fat-soluble vitamins, and providing a stronger immune system. It can also be used as an energy source, if needed. From a strictly weight loss point of view, they help you by making meals taste better, keeping you fuller for longer (extremely important while dieting, as you can imagine), and regulating blood sugars.

It's also worth noting that low-fat diets appear to affect our hormones in a negative way, most importantly testosterone levels (Dorgan et al., 1996, Hämäläinen et al., 1983, Volek et al., 1997). Low "T levels" are not something any male, especially one in his late 40's and upwards, would ever want. Low T levels will make it more difficult to get lean, build muscle, and improve your strength. So be sure to get some saturated fat into your diet (as opposed to just fat in general) as it's important for maintaining optimal testosterone levels (Volek et al., 1997).

Recommended dietary fat intake

Most general recommendations suggest that fat intake accounts for 20-30% of someone's total calories (Learney,

2015). I've never been a huge fan of using percentages for calculating someone's macronutrients, but these percentages equate fairly well to 0.48-0.72g of fat per kilo of bodyweight, and so that's how I calculate people's fat intakes for setting up a weight loss phase (McDonald, 2008).

> *Example (90kg man):*
> *Daily dietary fat intake: 90 x 0.48 - 0.72 = 43.2 - 64.8g*
> *Again, we would round it up or down so, 43-65g per day*

There are diets that go much higher. Ketogenic (very low to zero carb) diets, for example, have fat intakes as high as 75% of total calories, and there seem to be some benefits to this style of diet for health. I'm not an expert on keto diets because I would never want to eat such low carbs permanently, but if this interests you, I'd recommend a book by Lyle McDonald[7] called The Ketogenic Diet for more information.

Things to consider

For some of you, including fats into part of a healthy weight loss diet might be difficult at first, due to the many years you were told that this was bad for you. Therefore, don't be surprised if this lifestyle change feels a little odd in the beginning, and you find yourself questioning it. It usually becomes easier as you begin to feel the benefits.

We should discuss how you are going to choose your starting fat intake. If you look back at the example using a 90kg guy, there is quite a big difference between 45g and 63g of fat.

---

7 Lyle McDonald is an exercise physiologist and author renowned for being one of the top guys in sports nutrition, weight loss and research. He is someone whose advice and information I respect immensely.

Essentially, what you must remember is this: the more fat you choose to eat, the lower your carbs can be.

If you're someone who likes more carbs, trains more intensely, and/or has a very active job, then choose the lower end of the fat intake spectrum so you can squeeze in more carbs. Alternatively, some of you might prefer a diet higher in fat and therefore will opt for less carbs. Simply put, choose what you feel works best for you. Can you sense a theme here, yet?

Each gram of fat you consume will provide you with 9 calories. Just over double that of protein and carbs. Be aware of this. Overeating things like nuts, which is easily done, can really add up!

Carbohydrates – "So I can eat carbs even if I want to lose weight?"

Carbohydrates, without a doubt, are the most common macro to be cut out of a diet when someone is looking to lose some weight. That's because we have been scared shitless into believing that sugar is singlehandedly responsible for our obesity epidemic. I wonder how many of you reading this believe that you can't eat foods like bread and pasta if you want to be leaner. I'd bet my left nut that a large percentage of you do! In this section, I'll clear that myth up, and ensure that you understand how, and even why, you should include those delicious carbs into your diet – while still getting leaner. It's okay, no need to thank me, it's all part of the service.

The main role of carbs is that they provide our body with energy[8]. We get can get carbs from a number of sources, including veggies, grains, fruits and sugar, something that I'll discuss in more detail later on. Many of you will have

---

8 Although remember that the body can (and will) use fats and proteins as an energy source under certain circumstances.

a strange relationship with carbs; eating them in abundance when your weight isn't a priority, yet the minute you want to drop a few kilos, they're cut right out. As I've already said, this is because you'll consider them to be the reason you're overweight, making their removal an obvious choice.

The problem is many guys will feel like crap on a very low carb diet. A friend I was speaking to recently commented that his brother had lost a lot of weight a couple of years ago using a diet that completely eliminated carbs. He had even maintained that lifestyle for two long painful years even though he "hated it" and was "always miserable". Unfortunately for him, the fact that his diet was low in carbs wasn't what helped him lose weight. It was because he had maintained a calorie deficit. Had he known that, he could have a chosen a more enjoyable nutritional plan to follow. These stories are so painful to hear, but it's a mistake many of you will make, and just another reason why I've written this book.

Don't believe me? Well, one study (Johnston et al., 2006) concluded that when calories and protein are equated, there is no metabolic advantage (one won't cause more weight loss than the other) between ketogenic diets (carbs making up just 5% of total calories) and non-ketogenic diets (carbs making up 40% of total calories). In other words, the reason people lose weight is – drum roll, please – due to creating a calorie deficit, as we have already discussed. What most research shows, and something that I highly agree with through my own experience, is that there is no single "best" diet from a nutritional standpoint. The "best" diet is the one that you can stick to.

Recommended daily carb intake

We have already calculated your daily protein and fat

needs. Therefore, it should be fairly obvious that what is left of your calories will come from your carb choices. I feel that because protein and fat are so important, it's essential we ensure we have adequate calories for them first, before deciding what to use for carbs. Think of the calories used for protein and fat like the money you must have to cover your mortgage, petrol, bills, food and basic clothing. It's not until those are accounted for that you know what is left to be spent on leisure and luxuries.

We have already established that protein will provide you with 4 calories per gram, and fat provides 9 calories per gram. We also know what your total calories for the day are going to be, as well as how many grams of protein and fat you require. From here, we can simply calculate how many calories are left, and then equate that to grams of carbs. Carbs, like protein, provide you with 4 calories per gram.

Example:

Imagine that your recommended daily calories are 2500, your protein is 250g and your fat is 50g. Your plan would look like so:

1. Calories: 2500
2. Protein: 250 x 4 = 1000 calories
3. Fat: 50 x 9 = 450 calories
4. Calories from protein and fat: 1000 + 450 = 1450
5. Calories left for carbs: 2500 - 1450 = 1050
6. Carbs: 1050 / 4 = 262.5 (I'd round down to 260g)

Your plan will have 260g of carbs in it per day. Got it? Perfect, let's move on.

Consider these thoughts

Like with the protein, you can opt for a higher or lower amount of fat, and this of course affects the amount of carbs you can have without exceeding your calories. As fats increase, carbs have to go down, and vice versa. I suggest that you keep this bigger picture in mind when you are calculating your macros.

You have to remember that your carbs are your fuel, and just like a car, the more you move or the faster you go, the more fuel is required. If you spend a lot of time sat at your desk and the only real time you move is when you go to the gym, then you don't need as many carbs – therefore, you would opt for a higher fat, lower carb approach. On the other hand, if you are like my client Tim, who works in London and makes himself walk as much as possible, routinely averaging 17,000 steps per day (~8 miles!), then you will need more carbs. You also don't have to eat exactly the macros you have calculated. I've had clients get worried because they have exceeded their fats by 5g... yes, 5! Think of those numbers as guidelines and try to stay near to them, but don't overly stress over being exact. It will rarely happen! You now know that the most important factors for fat loss are the calories you eat and the protein you consume (and even that can vary a lot, if needed). After that all you really need is some fats for health and carbs to fuel your lifestyle. This gives you a ton of flexibility. This will be discussed in more detail later in the book.

There are some psychological issues to consider as well. Some of you will find that carbs tend to trigger cravings that increase the chances of you binging. If this is you, then don't opt for a higher carb approach. Similarly, don't choose a very low carb diet if it makes you feel like shit and leaves you struggling to exercise, run your business, and makes you so grumpy that your family wants to disown you. Find the sweet spot of being able to lose some weight and being able to sustain the plan for long enough to see some results without hating your life. Believe me, the people around you will thank you.

Finally, I know I will get a lot of resistance about that information, but that's fine; I expect it. As I've commented already, many of you will have it ingrained into your heads that you must embark on a low-carb diet in order to lose weight. Ironically (as well hilariously and stupidly), it's often the guys who will disagree with me that need the most help. It's strange that so many can become so attached to a certain dogma that they will continue to defend it even when it doesn't work. This would be like struggling to position your business well in your niche, asking for the advice of someone who's clearly an expert in premium positioning, and then telling them that their suggestions won't work. However, there are many guys who just find change difficult. I accept that. Be smart, and don't be one of them, please!

Do this NOW before reading on:

1. Calculate how many calories you require:
   BW (kg) x 22-26
2. Calculate your protein requirements:
   BW (kg) x 1.6-3.1
3. How many calories do you get from the protein:
   Protein (g) x 4
4. Calculate your fat requirements:
   BW (kg) x 0.48-0.72
5. How many calories do you get from the fat:
   fat (g) x 9
6. Add up the calories from protein and fat

7. Work out how many calories are left for carbs:
   Total calories - the answer from No.6
8. Convert those calories for carbs into grams of carbs:
   Calories for carbs / 4

Common dieting myths to ignore

"If I eat late at night, will it turn to fat?!"

I was doing some market research recently and found myself on a weight-loss forum. One post caught my eye, and as soon as I read it, I found myself thinking, "No wonder so many people struggle to lose weight". One guy had made a post that said (and I'm paraphrasing a little here), "I've decided to stop eating anything after 5pm. If I eat anything after that time, I find myself in the kitchen, raiding the fridge and binging". Now look, if that works for him, then great, and if you to want to try it as well, then so be it. I'm not saying you can't do this, but let's be honest, it's pretty extreme.

I believe that your diet should be as "normal" as possible, so that once it's over, nothing has to change too dramatically. Not eating after 5pm is certainly going to make things like eating with family, friends and having any form of social life almost impossible. I'd also be willing to bet that the reason that eating after 5pm makes him binge is because the rest of his diet is fucking awful. It wouldn't surprise me in the slightest if this guy was practically starving himself for most of the day, and eating his dinner was likely triggering his uncontrollable eating.

While I'm discussing the subject of not eating throughout the day, if any of you do this because you're "too busy" with work, and therefore forget to eat, then find yourself eating everything in sight in the evening, I would suggest you address this quickly. This issue often boils down to two things. One is not being organised and having meals to eat, and therefore feeling like you don't have the time to go and get something. This problem is obviously solved by ensuring that you have some prepared meals with you at all times. It can be something as simple as a protein shake and a bag of nuts. The second issue is that eating frequently just isn't a habit. If you've got into the habit of missing meals for a long time, then this will be just be something you're used to.

You might also be interested to know that the hormone responsible for hunger, Ghrelin, gets used to the number of meals you eat per day, and therefore will be released at the times you are usually eating. If you drop down to, say 2 meals a day, after a short period of time, you will, in theory, only get hungry twice a day, at those times. It consequently makes sense that after a while, you wouldn't even experience hunger to remind you that you should eat. This can be overcome in the early days by setting alarms to remind you to eat. If you do this consistently over several weeks, you should get to the point where you are stopping to have some food.

Moving on from that poor guy, remember that there are actual people out there who will ADVISE that you stop eating food at a certain time. More common, though, is the recommendation that you shouldn't eat carbs late at night because "you'll store them as fat as you are inactive" – this is total bollocks. In fact, many of my clients eat some carbs at night because carbs will release the hormone serotonin and it helps them sleep. Perfect for those who don't find it easy to relax and sleep after a busy day. This never hinders their fat loss, ever. It's mad that this kind of information is still being touted as diet advice.

"I rarely eat breakfast, and I know that isn't helping me lose weight."

Another piece of advice that gets thrown around a lot is that you must eat breakfast in order to lose weight. Again, utter nonsense. One 16-week study showed that regardless of whether the participants ate breakfast or skipped it, there was no real difference in their body fat percentage at the end (Dhurandhar et al., 2014). Personally, I actually like to wait a few hours before I eat my first meal. This is also convenient, as it provides time to get some work or cardio done.

Another benefit of doing this while dieting is that it pushes all your meals closer together, and this tends to help you feel fuller throughout the day. When your calories get low, the last thing you want to be doing is spreading them over a 15- or 16-hour day. It provides a psychological benefit as well, because your last meal gets pushed to a later time at night. For most people, the evening will be the harder time to maintain willpower, because hunger is high, other people might be eating around you, and we tend to associate relaxation with food. When was the last time you watched a film or some sports and didn't want something to snack on?

When it comes to the question of whether or not you should eat breakfast, the answer really depends on how that choice affects you. As with skipping meals during the day, for some of you, skipping breakfast can lead to overeating later in the day. Again, choose the option that makes sticking to your plan the easiest. Don't skip breakfast if you find that several hours later, you're so hungry you can't control what you eat.

If you're someone who struggles with a poor appetite, then you might want to eat first thing in the morning so that you have plenty of time throughout the rest of the day to eat all your food. This especially goes to those of you that have higher calorie (and most likely higher protein) demands. Spacing your meals out more may make them easier to eat.

Play around with this, but once again, I'll remind you that the most important factor for fat loss is eating the correct number of calories each day, consistently. This means that missing breakfast is okay as long as it doesn't affect how much you eat over the course of the whole day.

"If I eat lots of little meals, it speeds up my metabolism, right?"

Traditionally, people tend to believe the old myth that eating lots of smaller meals throughout the day will help them lose weight quicker. The conventional wisdom is that this will speed up your metabolism. Unfortunately, this is not actually the case (Bellisle, McDevitt and Prentice, 1997). Like many of the diet myths out there that aren't true, if you listen to them, they can actually make dieting much, much harder.

I'll clear this issue up by explaining that eating a meal does slightly and temporarily increase your metabolism. We know this already. The problem is that how much your metabolism increases is directly proportional to the size of the meal you eat. If you ate 3 big meals in a day, you would get 3 large rises in metabolism. If you ate 6 smaller meals per day you, would get 6 smaller rises in your metabolism. However, all other things being equal, those "rises" will ultimately be the same, whether they are comprised of six small rises or three large ones. In other words, the weight loss would be no different, because they will both burn the same number of calories.

Now that we know that eating frequent, smaller meals won't help you lose more body fat, we can discuss why knowing this is important for you. Once again, it simply comes down to your ability to be able to consistently stick to your plan – by now, I'm sure you knew that was coming, right? As I've stated several times, you need your diet plan to fit into your life the best that it can. You shouldn't have to fit your life into the plan, within reason. By all means, you can certainly try, but I guarantee you won't last long.

A few years ago, I had a very busy client who was adamant that he needed 7 meals per day. I can't remember where he had read this, but he had got it from somewhere, and I couldn't do anything to convince him otherwise. The issue was that due to his hectic life – running a business and having 3 children to contend with – he'd usually only manage three to four meals, at best. On several occasions, I suggested that he would be better served by spreading his calories across three to four meals, and every time he shot me down with, "No, I will just get better at eating all of my meals".

The problem was that he was never able to accomplish this, and it resulted in a number of failures, lots of frustration, and, in the end, shitty results. I did warn him. His failure came purely as a result of his belief that something he had read was how it must be done, and being unable to let go of that. It probably had more to do with his ego, to be honest. He was an arrogant twat and didn't like being told he was wrong (I'm assuming he wasn't used to it). I still wonder why the fuck he paid me in the first place. It's worth mentioning that in fitness and health, there is rarely just one way to do something. If someone explains things to you in absolutes, I'd steer clear of their advice.

The take-home point here is that you really need to choose the number of meals you eat each day based on making the diet as simple for you to follow as possible. I've just briefly discussed the issue of actually being able to eat the meals you've prepared yourself, but there some other factors to consider as well.

You also need to consider how the meal frequency you choose affects your hunger. Some people will find that eating a few large meals can actually cause them to binge in between them, as the lengths of time between meals are larger. I've had clients who have opted for more frequent meals, and this made them want to overeat as well. Choosing the amount of meals that makes it easiest to stick to your calorie allowance is your priority.

Appetite and meal size should also be considered. If you weigh 120kg and need 3100 calories, and opt to eat three meals per day, then you'll have to be able to eat meals that are just over a thousand calories. Is this going to be easy for you? Are those meals going to be too large? If you are so busy with work that you rarely stop to eat, are you really going to find the time to eat a large meal? You might be better with several smaller meals that you can eat in 5-10 minutes and be back to work. Similarly, if you are 60kg and only require ~1400 calories, you might find that breaking them up into six servings of roughly 230 leaves you feeling hungry. Plus, it's more of a pain in the arse preparing six little meals, all in their own containers. When you consider meal frequency, think about the size of the meals you'd prefer. Essentially, what we are keen to ensure is that the number of meals you choose feels the best to you and is easily implemented into your day-to-day routine.

At the risk of contradicting myself a little, I do have a recommendation on the minimum number of meals you should aim for each day, where possible. That recommendation would be to aim to eat three meals per day. Although there may be no metabolic advantage to eating smaller meals for your metabolism, there is one reason why it would be more optimal to eat at least eat three meals per day. That is the need to supply the body with regular servings of protein to help ensure that you maintain muscle throughout the diet. As Brad Schoenfeld[9] suggests, the muscle building effects of a meal last "…a maximum of six hours or so. Thus, consumption of at least three meals spaced out every five to six hours would seem to be optimal" to maintain muscle (Schoenfeld, 2017). Knowing that you can choose between three and six meals per day also gives you plenty of flexibility, because you know that you have some leeway to play with. Again, this is just more diet flexibility that allows you to plan your diet around your day.

From a practical point of view, you also must remember that protein isn't that easy to eat, as I've already discussed. This is a good thing for feeling full, but I've had clients who have needed 300g of protein per day try to consume all 300g in just 3 meals. 100g of protein in a single meal will be very tough for some of you to eat. That is the equivalent of roughly 400g of uncooked lean meat. That is a fair amount, believe me. The most I tend to have per meal is 200g of uncooked lean meat. Bear all this in mind when you are creating your plan. I don't really feel there is any need to go over six meals per day unless that is your preference, or you simply need that many meals to make the calories manageable.

Before we move on, I feel I had better say that there will be the odd day where you do only eat a couple of meals. You might be busier than usual, or something just comes up that messes with your plans. That's life, it happens. Don't freak out. Remember, it's what you do consistently that counts, and the odd day like this will not mess anything up. I don't want any of you worrying because I suggested aiming for three to six meals and you only managed two on a handful of

---

9   Brad Schoenfeld is a renowned trainer, author, and researcher in the field of fitness and nutrition. He is involved in a lot of the current research being done.

occasions over the course of 12 weeks. This really goes for everything you read in this entire book. 80% on track for a lifetime beats 100% on track for a few weeks.

Daily tracking - being accountable leads to success

I find that people are more successful when they accurately track what foods and drinks they're consuming on a day-to-day basis, at least during times of dieting. I feel it is more effective for people to do this by tracking their daily macronutrients and their calories, rather than something more subjective like portion sizes, at least the majority of the time. There will, of course, be times when you'll be required to "eyeball" your food to ensure you don't overeat, such as when eating in hotels and restaurants. Even then, though, many places will tell you their steak is 8oz, for example, or will provide the nutritional info online or on the menu, making it fairly easy, even in those situations, to stay on track if you're sensible.

I know many will say it's "obsessive", but it works, and it's a lot easier than you'd think. The issue that most people will have with tracking their food by eye is that they will often underestimate how much food they're eating. I did this once with the bowl of cereal I have after the gym. I needed 60g, and I weighed it out on three, maybe four occasions but then began to just pour them by eye. A few weeks later, I decided to weigh out what I was now believing to be 60g, and it turned out I was eating closer to 90g, which is a massive difference. Fortunately, at the time I wasn't dieting, but it was still an eye opener. In fact, you'll often find that people will underestimate their daily food intake (calories) by a massive 30%, with the range being somewhere between 10% and 45% depending on factors such as age and sex (Nestle, 2017). This is important, because if you're getting your daily intake wrong, it can make a huge difference to your results.

This seems insane, but having heard many people over the years say to me, "I can't seem to lose weight, even though I'm eating healthily", it doesn't surprise me. The common factor with almost all of them is that they have no idea what their daily calorie intake is (and importantly, what it even should be). In my opinion, tracking your food intake is extremely important for successful fat loss. Be prepared to purchase some weighing scales and learn to read food labels.

What we need to discuss, then, is a format in which you can do this easily. I'd recommend that you aim to weigh out and prepare meals at home to take with you during the day as often as possible. This gives you full control of what you put into your mouth. However, if you are busy running a business, there will be times where this is simply unrealistic, like at business meetings or when travelling.

One of my current clients, for example, is a couple of months into his plan. He has nailed it so far, and the changes he has made are amazing. Now, this phase has been relatively easy for him, as he's not been away at all the whole time. It's meant that he's been able to stick to his plan 100% and not have any real problems in doing so. This is about to change, as he will soon be leaving for a whole month of business travel. That's one full month of hotels, airports, not knowing where the gym is, eating out, etc. That will definitely prove to be much harder for him to follow the plan. It obviously means there will be times when he literally can't prepare his food like he usually would.

This will not be a problem, as we have a solution for this which I'll explain to you now. Without a solution for these specific times, many of you would use it as an excuse to not follow your plan; you'd say you had "no option". But this need not be the case.

Before we talk about how to go about tracking your food during times like these, please remember that just because there might be things such as biscuits and alcohol on offer at certain events that you attend, that doesn't mean you have to eat them. You always have a choice. What I'm saying, then, is that at times, you will need to have some self-control. This should be obvious, but I know what it's like to be on a diet; and in these situations, your brain will want to screw you over at every possible moment. Man up and stay in control.

Now, let's assume that you do have some self-control and are focused on achieving your goals, but you are in a situation where you need to order something that you might usually consider "bad", like a large plate of pasta, for example. Most of you will believe that this meal will ruin everything. Chances are that you would just say "Fuck it" and forget about your goal; leading to the infamous "I'll start again Monday" mentality. But it certainly doesn't have to be this way! There really is no need to worry. All you need to do is ensure that you just track the meal and account for it.

In the previous chapters, you should have calculated how many calories per day you require, and of course how many grams of protein, carbs, and fats, as well. And because you know this information, having the large plate of pasta we discussed above is fine, as long as you don't go over the calories for the day. You can think of your daily calories as being like a budget. This is a budget you must look at each day, and so long as you keep track of what you are spending your "money" on, you're fine.

Think of the protein as the most important things to buy, such as petrol to fuel your car. You must ensure that you save enough of the total budget to meet your needs for the day. Understanding this allows you to fit certain meals into your plan on days where it might be a little less predictable, or you can't eat prepared meals.

The best way to do this is with your mobile phone or laptop using an app like MyFitnessPal (MFP). Free apps for your phone like MFP are great. You can enter the foods you have eaten into the app, and it will track this over the course of days, weeks, and months. At the touch of a button, you can see how many calories you've eaten; and, perhaps more importantly, how many you have left. It's like being able to check your bank balance to ensure you don't end up in the red. The great thing about some of these apps is that you can enter the data of your meal manually, scan barcodes from products, or search a pretty extensive database of foods, brands, and restaurants. This, in my opinion, makes the job of daily accountability simple and easy.

Another very important reason for tracking your food intake is that it allows you to easily adjust the plan when progress starts to stall (which it will at some point!). In business articles and speaking to clients, I've heard this said many times[10]: "What gets measured gets managed". This couldn't be more true for achieving your fitness goals as well!

If you've been tracking and measuring your food by "eye", then it's fairly difficult to then be able to reduce the number of your calories in a controlled manner, with any real accuracy. If you are the person whose diet plan would usually consist of "cutting out junk" and you're not tracking anything at all, then this becomes impossible. I'll say it again – what gets measured gets managed, and if you can't manage your plan, then you're screwed.

Instead, why not just take a little time to weigh out your food? This way, when the time comes, it can be easily reduced,

---

10   Apparently, this was said by Peter Drucker, although a search for a source found many different versions of the quote, as well as several different origins. Whatever, it's still a great quote!

and with accuracy. For example, reducing your pasta serving from 150g to 100g is far easier than trying to change the serving size, and allows you to assess the outcome (do you lose more weight or not) and decide if the changes you made were sufficient. I'm going to cover exactly how to make calorie adjustments later in the book.

One last reason to track is simply this: people forget what they've eaten.

I know this sounds stupid, but all it takes is a busy day or a sleepless night, and you can easily begin to wonder what you've eaten that day.

Believe me when I say that most times, you'll come to the conclusion that you've not eaten a meal so that you have a reason to eat more food. Again, I'll say it: your brain is going to fuck with you quite a bit in an attempt to stop you losing weight. Don't risk it.

The only downside

The only small downside to using something like a food tracking app is that their databases may not always be 100% accurate. Some apps like MyFitnessPal, for example, actually allow their users to enter food data into the database. You can imagine the issue with this, right? The good apps will often have entries that are "verified," but I think it's worth knowing this. Personally, I don't think that it's a big issue. Even the food labels you get on the foods aren't always all that accurate. The thing is, consistency always wins. If you're using the same maths day in and day out for a certain food or product, then it doesn't really matter if the calories are slightly off, because you'll be eating the same amount of it each time. If that amount doesn't lead to progress, then you'll simply reduce the amount of it you eat.

What I tend to do if using an app is cross reference the

nutritional info it provides me with the nutritional info provided by a product's own website, just to see if they match up. For generic things like potatoes, blueberries, rice and chicken that really don't vary that much, I just use the same maths every time, regardless of the brands of the product.

Do this NOW before reading on:

1. Go to www.myfitnesspal.com and download the app or find one similar.

The "all or nothing dieting" mentality

I talk about something I call the "all or nothing dieting mentality" a lot with clients and in my writing, and for good reason. It's important to consider, if you want results that will last you a lifetime.

Humans seem to love extremes, and the way in which most people eat and drink is no different. What I mean by an "all or nothing dieting mentality" is that most people will sit perfectly at one of the two extreme ends of a dieting spectrum for much of their lives:

1. They are not currently dieting. This is reflected by poor food choices and a total lack of self-control when it comes to portion sizes. This means that their overall daily calorie consumption is well above what they require. They take a very relaxed attitude towards their wellbeing and overall health.

2. They are trying to improve their health, fitness, and lose some flab. They're extreme, cutting calories very low, which leads to hunger and cravings. More often than not, certain foods and macronutrients are completely cut out (sugar probably being the best example), because they believe they are "bad" and

will stop them losing weight. They become overly obsessed by the notion of "being on a diet" and this often becomes a very consuming part of their lives, much to their detriment.

Rarely will people find the middle ground of that spectrum. One day, it's a shitty diet of microwave meals, takeaways, hotel desserts, and beer; the next, it's grilled chicken, rice and steamed veg. They move from one extreme to the next. I'm fairly confident that you're not a bodybuilder or professional athlete, nor do you have any aspirations of being one. You do not have to follow a diet like one because your goals are far more modest. Bodybuilders and athletes will often follow a diet that's referred to as a "clean". "Clean" foods tend to be seen as the ones that are the healthiest because they're natural, unrefined and unprocessed. Vegetables, chicken breast, and extra virgin olive oil are all examples of foods considered to be "clean". "Dirty" foods, on the other hand, are those that are highly processed, fatty, and low in vitamins and minerals; for example, chocolate bars, crisps, and pizza. These so-called "dirty" foods tend to be off-limits for much of the diet, unless they're having a "cheat meal" (we'll cover cheat meals in another section).

Now, the issue with following a strict "clean diet" is that most of you just won't be able to sustain it for more than a few weeks, at best. It's boring and extremely restrictive. When diet choices like this are made, it's only a matter of time before the dieter has what I call the "fuck it" moment, where they can't carry on any longer and decide to give up. Obviously, after such a restrictive diet, all they'll want to do is eat the foods they've missed and return to their old, normal diet. The only outcome here is rapid weight regain, and feeling pissed off with yourself for failing.

Trying to follow a diet plan that is overly restrictive and

boring is not the kind of diet that is going to help you if you want to stay fit, healthy and look great long-term. You require a diet plan that easily fits into your life with minimal disruption. We only have to look at dieting statistics and at the people around us to see that the more "traditional" extreme mentality to dieting isn't fucking working! Strangely, there are still many personal trainers, coaches, and even doctors who will prescribe diets of this nature. For personal trainers, this is often because it's all they know. Some just believe that everyone needs to be "hardcore". They are stupid and wrong, and if you ever receive a diet plan that resembles something like this, then get your money back and walk away. Success lies somewhere in the middle of this spectrum. The diagram below summarises this well:

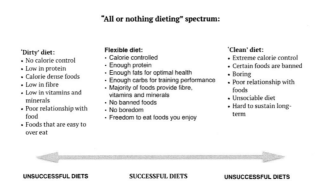

"All or nothing dieting" spectrum:

'Dirty' diet:	Flexible diet:	'Clean' diet:
• No calorie control	• Calorie controlled	• Extreme calorie control
• Low in protein	• Enough protein	• Certain foods are banned
• Calorie dense foods	• Enough fats for optimal health	• Boring
• Low in fibre	• Enough carbs for training performance	• Poor relationship with foods
• Low in vitamins and minerals	• Majority of foods provide fibre, vitamins and minerals	• Unsociable diet
• Poor relationship with food	• No banned foods	• Hard to sustain long-term
• Foods that are easy to over eat	• No boredom	
	• Freedom to eat foods you enjoy	

UNSUCCESSFUL DIETS   **SUCCESSFUL DIETS**   **UNSUCCESSFUL DIETS**

I've found that my clients get far greater results when they are allowed some flexibility within their diets. This is often aptly referred to simply as "flexible dieting", but really, it's just remembering the old cliché that with food and drink, "everything in moderation" is fine. It's hardly surprising, though, that having the freedom to consume the foods and drinks you enjoy (albeit in moderation) makes following a diet far, far easier. In fact, at this point, I'm reluctant to even call it a "diet" anymore, because I feel this is where we can describe what you're doing as simply following a "lifestyle" that's designed to help you lose weight.

As I've discussed in other chapters, the most important thing to get right while dieting is consuming the right number of calories and grams of protein. If you meet those needs while getting a good amount of healthy fats, then enjoying something you might normally feel is "bad" won't hurt your progress. The key to enjoying a more flexible diet approach is to remember to choose foods that fill you up as much as possible without triggering binges. This is vitally important. For example, I certainly know that if I have something like chocolate, I rarely feel satisfied. In fact, it actually makes me crave more, often actually worse than the original craving I'd had before it was eaten.

Broadly speaking, we could compare this to an alcoholic trying to have a glass of wine now and again. It simply doesn't work. Although I'm definitely not suggesting you are addicted to certain foods, what I am saying is that some foods will make the diet harder to stick to. Yes, some flexibility is great, but only if it doesn't actually make your diet more difficult. This is something you'll have to find out yourself through experience, over time, and some trial and error. The reward for doing so will be the ability to create diet plans that are easy to stick to for long enough to get results, and that does not lead to binges after the diet is over because you have not felt restricted throughout the process. Remember that the diet that's best for you is the one you can follow for long enough to get some bloody results.

How to properly track your progress – "Do I really have to send you photos, Phil?"

In this section, I'm going to teach you how you should go about actually tracking your progress on a weekly basis, thus ensuring that you know that what you're doing is working, and if it isn't, when to make changes to your plan. This is something that will be covered in great detail later on.

I'm hoping this section will also clear up the issue of using weighing scales for tracking once and for all, because quite frankly, it gets tiring answering the same questions on it. The weight people see on the scales leads to so much confusion, frustration, and grief that it's definitely something I need to address. For most, the scale weight will be placed on some kind of weight loss pedestal, where for some reason, it receives way too much value. I've had clients actually check in with a reduction in their body measurements but will report feeling unhappy because their weight on the scale hadn't changed. I told you dieting will mess with your brain! But by the end of this section, you'll see why this is not something that should cause you any worry.

Let's remember that weight on the scale isn't a true representation of overall body fat. The weight you see is the combination of bone, skin, muscle, food, water, et cetera, and therefore can be an unreliable tool for tracking progress if used on its own. I had one guy recently complaining all week that he wasn't feeling well and that his weight wasn't going down. What he failed to understand was that his weight wasn't going down due to water retention being caused by being unwell. When his weekly "check-in" came, he was about 1kg heavier than the previous week. I knew this would be the case due to his bug, but what was still shocking to him was that his weekly photos were showing that he had still made some great progress when compared with the previous week. This example proves the importance of using multiple tracking tools.

Another reason you have to be careful with using just the weight on the scale is that those of you who are new (or returning after a long break) to weight training will often gain a little muscle in the first several weeks, even though you're dieting. Therefore, total weight loss will often be far less than you'd expect. My client Jon is a great example of this. See the photo below:

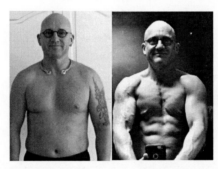

Clearly, you can see that Jon's body fat is remarkably lower. What's fascinating is that the weight difference here was, in fact, only 3kg (6.6lbs).

If you look closely, though, you'll see why. Look at the difference in the size of his shoulders, arms and chest. The weight of that newly gained muscle offsets the weight of the fat lost. This, in fact, is the ideal scenario. Losing fat while gaining some muscle, leaving a well-defined physique at the end, is the "holy grail" of dieting. Oh, and Jon was about four weeks from being 52 at the time. Yes, it can be done at any age.

What I'm saying is that, in the short term, the scales aren't usually a very reliable tracking tool. This is often due to the water retention caused by dieting than anything else. When we diet, we tend to hold more water due to hormonal changes. Bear in mind that it's not uncommon to hold so much water that it essentially hides any fat loss from being "seen" on the scales. If you lose 0.5kg of fat, but have 1kg of extra water at the end of the week, you're going to feel disappointed if you don't take this into consideration.

Let's look at the options for tracking your progress. Here is a list of the best tracking tools and some considerations:

Weighing scales (for a fasted weight)

I've already covered the weighing scales a little and discussed their limitations; however, they are still a very valuable tool that I recommend using. In the short term, like over 1-10 days, they can often not show much in the way of progress. But in the long term, over weeks and months, they are a great tool for tracking your progress. For most, it doesn't matter how much water you hold or muscle you build, the scales will show a downward trend over the long term, especially for those of you with more body fat to lose.

Here is a case study that proves my point, using my client Mark's progress. Firstly, let's look at the difference in the amount of body fat he displays around his love handles and back from his start photo to week 9:

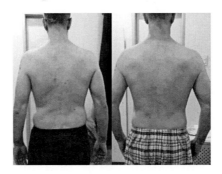

It should be fairly clear that his body fat has reduced. So now let's look at the graph of his weight over that same time period (9 weeks, remember):

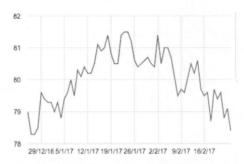

There we have it. He started his diet on Christmas Eve (no, seriously!) at a weight of 79kg, and didn't return to that weight for about nine weeks! Every week, his photos were showing he had less and less fat, but as you can see from the graph, his weight was actually rising. At one point, it was up by around 2.5kg. What I'm saying is that you shouldn't rely on just the scales, and certainly shouldn't be quick to believe that you are failing if your weight actually begins to increase in the beginning.

Remember to weigh yourself fasted in the morning after you have been to the bathroom, as this will make the weight as reliable and as consistent as possible. From a purely tracking point of view, I have my client check in with their weight every 7 days. However, if we are talking about accountability, weighing yourself daily might be a solid plan of action. Recent research has found that people who weigh themselves more frequently, even every day, actually lose more weight (and regained less after) than those who didn't (Linde et al., 2005, VanWormer et al., 2011). I do this personally, as I like to just keep an eye on the way things are going. I would imagine this works because you know that you're going to "see" your weight every morning, and this is enough to deter some people from consuming extra calories the day before.

For some of you, this might actually cause more stress than it's worth, because seeing the daily fluctuations will cause concern. Just remember, they are only changes in water weight and not fat. I suggest you choose an option that suits your personality. Do not, however, bury your head in the sand and totally avoid weighing yourself at all. I've had many clients do so over the years because they're fearful that they've not lost weight. Get yourself on that scale and make yourself accountable. If you've not been sticking to your plan and aren't progressing well, then tough shit. Deal with it and work out why you're failing to do so.

Photos

As a tool for tracking progress, the photograph is probably my favourite. You've already seen two examples where I've had to use photos to track a client's progress, as their weight alone was not sufficient to paint an accurate picture of their progress, and so it's probably pretty clear why I think they are such a great tool. I think that for most men, taking photos at the start can be pretty motivating. It's common for clients to comment that they hadn't "realised" they were actually that fat. It's often a shock to them, and this usually gets them in the mood to make some changes. The great thing about photos is that they provide a much better idea of what's happening with regards to the overall physique than just the numbers from the scale or body measurements. Over time, you'll see more definition and more muscle appear. This is usually the most motivating of all the ways in which you can track your progress. And if this is happening in a client's progress photos, then I don't give a shit about what the scales are saying that week. I tend to have clients send me photos every two weeks so that there is enough of a difference that it can be seen.

Bear in mind that in the beginning, you might not see much progress when you compare photos. If you have 15-20kg to lose, then let's be honest: losing 0.5-1kg isn't going to be easily noticeable. As you get leaner and more defined, your photos will actually show a great deal more progress, because your weekly fat loss begins to represent a larger percentage of your overall fat. That is the point where photos are really exceptional and highly rewarding. At this point, I'm inclined to suggest taking photos weekly, because progress will be very noticeable.

One tip I have when comparing your photos is not to concentrate on the areas that hold the most fat. As a man, that tends to be your abs, love handles, and lower back. The reason I say this is because the fat in those areas is often far more stubborn, and will therefore take longer to lean out. If you only look at those areas, there is a good chance you'll miss what's going on elsewhere on your body, as areas like arms, shoulders, and chest will usually lean out much faster. Be sure to take a look at these areas, too. This is also why I recommend you take photos from the front, the back and the side. The back is very important, as it's an area that you will rarely see for yourself! You will often be surprised about how much progress is going on back there that you hadn't noticed.

Calipers

For those who don't know, calipers are used to measure body fat in certain areas on your body in millimetres. Those readings can then be used to calculate a rough body fat percentage. Personally, I don't tend to calculate the body fat percentage, instead favouring to just record the individual readings that I've tested. It means that you can see how the body fat from different areas is progressing. For example, your records might resemble the table below:

Measurement in mm	Week 1	Week 2	Week 3	Week 4
Tricep	20mm	18mm	16mm	16mm
Bicep	10mm	9mm	8mm	8mm
Hip	25mm	25mm	23mm	23mm
Upper back	18mm	17mm	14mm	14mm
Total	73mm	69mm	61mm	61mm

Notice how from week 3 to week 4 there is no change in any of the readings. This would indicate that you may need to make some adjustments to your plan, to ensure you continue to make progress. I'd recommend you find a local coach or trainer that's good at this, as it does take practice. Be certain to use the same person consistently so the readings stay accurate. This is one of those tools that can vary a lot simply by asking a different person to help you. Caliper testing will also be affected by water retention, so if you do get readings that are similar to the previous week (like the table shows), then you will have to decide on whether you think it's a water issue or you genuinely haven't made any progress. Personally, I stopped using these once all of my work moved to online coaching. Asking clients to get calliper testing done just wasn't worth their time when I could see progress from other methods just as well. Nonetheless, it is a decent option.

Measurements

This is fairly self-explanatory. Take several measurements from places like your hips, waist, midsection, chest, arms, and thighs, and record them. Repeat this process every week to see how they're progressing. This is a good one, as your measurements will often shrink even if your weight remains the same. This is simply because fat is less dense than muscle. As with the table in the calliper testing section, you can simply input those weekly readings into a spreadsheet and keep a close eye on them.

Clothing

Whether it's general clothing you wear frequently or something that is currently too small, your clothes are a great indicator of progress. I hear this almost weekly: "Weight isn't down much, but clothes are fitting much looser". Something that many of my clients do is actually buy an item of clothing that won't fit, such as a pair of jeans with a waist size they're looking to achieve in the next few months. This can also serve as motivation as they begin to fit better and better over the course of the weeks. Just be sure to be realistic with how much smaller the clothing is. Those are the ones I tend to use most often. I don't use how clothing fits as a formal tool, merely as something that clients will observe over time. It's more of a bonus, to be honest.

In summary

Personally, I tend to rely predominantly on a person's fasted weight, their photos, and their measurements. The point is that you can't rely on one tool to do this, and you definitely don't go just by the scales.

Let me remind why you're tracking your progress in the first place: so that you're confident that your current plan of action is working.

Of course, it's great to see your physique changing over time, and this is very important, but the information you get from tracking simply answers this one question for you: "Is my plan working right now?". This is an important bit of information, because it allows you to decide on whether your plan needs to be adjusted or left the hell alone. We will cover diet adjustments in the next section, just so you know exactly what to do once progress does stall.

Making adjustments - "My progress has stopped! What do I do now?"

As I stated in the last chapter on tracking progress, one of the main reasons for tracking your progress is so that you can be confident that what you are doing is working. It also ensures that when the frustrating time comes that you aren't seeing any changes, that you can easily make the adjustments needed to get things moving again. It's no different from a successful marketing campaign going from getting plenty of quality, targeted leads to maybe a dribble; or worse, none at all. Fortunately, like with any marketing campaign, you can easily change your diet plan to ensure that progress doesn't stall for too long.

It's worth remembering that every diet plan will stop working, eventually, as the body begins to adapt to the number of calories that you're taking in and the training you're doing. In simple terms, the calorie deficit you initially created will eventually become a calorie balance, as the body fights against your attempts to lose weight. Therefore, it's obvious that in order to establish that calorie deficit again, adjustments to your plan must be made. You just need to keep an eye on when.

I want to discuss the "when" briefly now before going into the "how," because it's so important. Something to consider is that, unlike with business, during a diet, there are only a finite amount of changes that you can make to stop yourself from plateauing. There is only so much training and cardio that your body can recover from, and there certainly is a limit to how much you can reduce your food intake, before you're left with no more options.

I made this mistake the first time I ever made a diet plan for someone who was doing a fitness competition, where body fat levels have to be fairly low. Basically, I failed to correctly track the client's progress as well as I should have, using mostly the scale as my main tool. I didn't take into account that her physique was changing some weeks, even though her weight wasn't, and this led to me making the huge mistake of making changes to the plan far too frequently. What eventually happened was the client was still holding too much fat, but was also down to ~900 calories per day, and was doing a lot of cardio. In other words, I'd fucked it because I was out of options.

Luckily, we had started the diet very early to allow for mistakes like these, and therefore I had enough time to give her a full two-week diet break to get her metabolism fired up again. This allowed her to make much faster progress after we started dieting again. She went on to place 5th out of 34 girls – not too shabby – but that could have gone a lot worse. It's a very easy mistake to make, and therefore is very common. Please read this chapter carefully so you don't do the same.

Clearly, then, it's vital that you use your options carefully. As my mentor Ken "Skip" Hill [11] always says (and as I said in the previous chapter), "If it ain't broke, don't fix it". I've had clients (lucky ones) go 9-10 weeks without a single change. Lucky bastards! Then there are guys like me, who will feel like our bodies never want us to look lean, and so must make

11 Skip is a very well-established nutrition coach from the States, who has been coaching people in bodybuilding (as well as pros in sports like NFL) for 20 years or more. I was lucky enough to be chosen by him to be part of his mentorship programme. I've learnt so much from him! It was a worthy investment!

changes every couple of weeks. The goal is to "milk" your plan each time for all it's worth. Remember that.

What do we do if we don't see any progress from our tracking? Well, now I'll let you change something. First, though, I would always err on the side of caution, especially if you've plenty of time to achieve your goal. Yes, I'll make clients check in weekly, but it isn't uncommon for me to have them wait another three to seven days before we make any changes, especially if I believe that they are making progress toward their goals, but that progress is being hidden by water retention. If you don't get changes after a maximum of two weeks, then it's definitely time to adjust the diet.

So what changes should you make?

Remember that if you stop making progress, it just means that the body has created "balance" with your current plan. You're no longer using more calories than you're taking in, simple as that. We have two options for correcting this:

1. You can reduce the number of calories you're consuming.
2. You can increase the amount of exercise you are doing, and thus burn more calories per day, usually in the form of cardiovascular exercise.

Technically, you could use the third option, and decide to change both calories consumed and calories burned. However, personally, I'd suggest that you keep things simple and change one variable at a time: either eat less food, or do more exercise. The more control you have over these variables, the easier it is to measure the outcome. Now, let's look at these options in more detail.

Reducing your daily calorie intake

This really does not need to be overly complicated at all. When I want to reduce a client's calorie intake, I'll usually go with a 5-10% reduction.

> *Example:*
> *If you're consuming 2500 calories per day, then this would reduce to between 2250 and 2375*
> *2500 x 0.95 = 2374*
> *2500 x 0.9 = 2250*

I usually make my decision based on their progress. If someone hasn't made any progress at all, I'll go with the larger drop. If someone made some progress, albeit small, and just needs a small push in the right direction, then 5% will usually suffice. Again, I would err on the side of caution most of the time. You also should consider how many calories you're currently consuming. If you've already been dieting for a while, and may have already made several adjustments (meaning your calories could be fairly low), I would encourage you to make small adjustments.

Something to consider is where to take those calories from: protein, fats, or carbs. You should aim to keep your intake of protein and fat as high as possible, for reasons we have discussed previously, and so this leaves your carbs as the main macro that will get reduced when your diet plan changes. A combination of both could be considered if you have chosen to have your fat intake at the higher end at the start of the diet, as you have some to play with.

For those of you doing sports, longer cardio sessions, gym sessions with lots of sets, or have very active lifestyles in general, then aim to keep the carbs higher. If, like many people, you're fairly inactive, except for the training you've recently added in, then you can probably get away with lowering the carbs. I don't feel that many people need to be lower than 50g of carbs per day. That's not taken from any study, but simply from years of experience. Even that is fairly low for many people, but this would of course be relative to other factors, such as your body weight, as discussed in previous chapters.

At the end of the day, there is nothing that says you can't experiment. For many of you reading this, you will have to do a little trial and error to discover what you believe works the best for you. Remember, at the end of the day, you're just aiming to get back into a calorie deficit, so just reducing the calories will work, whether it's from the fats or the carbs. What you want to ensure is that you have enough energy to still function well at work, have energy for the children, and to feel good in the gym.

Choosing to do more exercise

You could simply burn more calories per day instead of reducing your food intake. This would have the same desired outcome, and could be accomplished by doing more weight training or more aerobic (cardio) training, whether that's in the gym or through a sport or activity you enjoy.

As with the reduction of calories, it's best to not be too aggressive with the changes. Do as little as you can to get the most results with everything fitness related. There are so many options and so many things to take into consideration when it comes to ramping up your cardio that it's difficult for me to give a very specific, black and white answer for how you should endeavour to increase it. However, that doesn't mean it's necessarily complicated to do it yourself! Here are some general rules I tend to abide by, the majority of the time.

Firstly, I think it is generally preferable for people to

increase the number of sessions they are doing per week before increasing the duration of their exercise. For example, if you were currently doing 2 x 20-minute sessions on a treadmill per week, you could change that to 2 x 30 minutes. However, my preference would be that you complete 3 x 20-minute sessions instead. You would then observe what results you get from that change and go from there.

Secondly, I prefer not to increase someone's cardio by more than 10 minutes per session if possible. The reason for this is that if you change the duration of your sessions from 30 minutes to say, 50 minutes, you'll never know if 40 minutes would have been sufficient. Remember, you're trying to always do the least amount possible while still getting the results you desire. Essentially, you want the best ROI that you can get for your time and energy.

One thing I'll add here is that unless you're doing endurance training because it's required, such as for a marathon or a similar endeavour, then I do not believe you will ever need to take your cardio training over 60 minutes in a single session. This really won't support the goal of getting stronger and maintaining muscle.

In the real world, those parameters above simply might not work for you. Let's assume you can only find time to make it to the gym three times per week. In that case, you don't have the option of going more frequently. This will likely force you to increase the duration of your cardio (I still wouldn't increase it by more than 10 minutes at a time, however). You may well in fact end up doing 3 x 60-minute sessions, instead of 6 x 30 minutes. Again, this is why it's difficult to make recommendations. You will have to find a way of getting the job done that fits your schedule.

In all honesty, the best thing you could probably do is invest in something like a treadmill or an elliptical trainer to use at home. It will provide you with the opportunity to get some cardio done at a time when it's convenient to you; and in most cases, that's going to be before work in the AM, or late at night.

We are going to cover cardiovascular training in greater detail later in the book to help make this decision easier.

Food choices – "So what foods should I eat to lose weight?"

Two very common questions I have to answer for clients are "What shall I actually eat?" and "How do I create meals with healthier foods?", and therefore this is something I felt needed to be addressed in this book to ensure it had some practical use and wasn't just all information. Also, let's be honest: there is a whole host of articles published online and in magazines that claim certain foods are "superfoods" for weight loss, while others should be completely avoided. That really confuses people and again, as I've stated before in this book, just makes dieting seem more difficult than it really is.

We have already discussed that for fat loss, the main things to consider are calorie needs and protein intake, and that you should get a certain amount of fats per day, which will leave you with some carbs to fuel your general activity and training. We have also said that diets can have some flexibility in them to include foods you enjoy. With that being said, there are certainly foods that, without a doubt, should make up the bulk of your diet.

The foods here tend to provide the following benefits:

- Quality protein for muscle retention
- Quality essential fats
- Leave you feeling fuller for longer
- Provide adequate vitamins, minerals and fibre

- Maintain stable blood sugar levels to reduce excessive hunger

Below are what I believe are some of the best options to choose from for your protein, fats and carbs.

Recommended protein sources:

- Lean chicken and turkey breast
- Fish i.e. cod, tuna, salmon
- Lean beef mince (5% fat or less)
- Egg whites
- Whey protein
- Cottage cheese & low-fat cheeses
- Dairy
- Beef steak (aim for leaner cuts)
- Pea or brown rice protein powder
- Quinoa
- Greek yogurt

Recommended fat sources:

- Extra virgin olive oil
- Butter
- Nuts / Nut butters
- Seeds
- Flaxseed / flax oil
- Coconut oil
- Oily fish i.e. salmon
- Omega 3 supplements (fish oils)
- Avocado
- Egg yolk

Recommended carb sources

- Sweet potato

- White potato
- Porridge oats
- Wholemeal bread
- Wholemeal pasta
- Rice
- Beans (black, kidney, etc.)
- Fruits (especially berries)
- Vegetables
- Quinoa
- Pancakes, cereal, pop tarts, sweets, white toast with jam, sorbet (perfect after weight training)

Those lists above aren't exhaustive, of course, but you could do a lot worse than eating from them 80-90% of the time and then having things you enjoy the rest of the time. There is *plenty there.*

What you will have to get used to doing as much as possible is preparing meals using those foods. Now, at times when you're eating out for business, or even with friends or family, I would recommend still choosing foods from the list. When you're in a restaurant, you really can't go wrong with something like a steak and steamed veg. If you want more carbs, then have some rice, or even fries; but you will often have to be very careful with them due to the portion sizes, and because chances are they will be high in fat. I have a client who eats out two or three times daily. He's still managed to make amazing progress simply by being sensible with his choices and sticking to meals that include foods, where possible, from the lists above.

Having said all this, none of those are by any means "superfoods" that will help you lose weight faster and easier, as if by magic. It's still possible to over-eat them, especially the ones that are higher in fats (and therefore calories per gram), such as nuts and nut butter, so be mindful of those choices.

"How do I create meals with healthier foods?"

Now, onto the next question about creating meals with these foods. This is important to discuss, as it's something I believe most people don't consider, and it can make dieting harder. Most, if not all, of the diets I evaluate from clients will at some point state that they snacked on something like a piece of fruit, or a cereal bar; in other words, something that is high in carbs, and low in protein and fat. These meals are not ideal, because they do not fill people up very well. You also have to worry about the rise and fall in blood sugars, which may lead to hunger more quickly than a more "complete" or balanced meal.

I'm a big believer that wherever possible, your meals should always at least contain protein and some fats. Every meal you consume, regardless of whether it's large, like for a traditional breakfast, lunch, or dinner, or small, like a snack, should have some protein and fats in there. The combination of eating some protein and fats in a single meal will keep you fuller for longer, while providing enough protein to maintain muscle. Carbs can be added to meals as and when needed for energy, based on how many you have to use. Although, I think it's a great idea to include vegetables in as many meals as possible.

The only time I will eat protein and carbs in a meal without some fats is after weight training. I don't want the fats, because they can feel harder to digest after a hard training session.

The key to these meals during a diet is ensuring that they fill you up. Eating meals that don't fill you up well is asking for trouble. You all know what it's like trying to stay on a "diet" when you're very hungry, especially in the evening when you're tired and your willpower is at its lowest. This is the time where you will end up reaching for something you're craving like pizza, beer, or crisps. In the blink of an eye, you could easily ruin a whole day of dieting. This is also why you should never go shopping when you're hungry. It's torture, and your basket or trolley will probably end up being full of junk.

For practical purposes, below is a typical training day's diet for me while dieting. I warn you though, I'm fairly boring, and so I encourage you to take some time to do this for yourself.

Typical training day while dieting:

Meal 1:
2 scoops of mint flavoured whey protein with water and ice
Cashews or extra virgin olive oil
Greens drink

3 hours later

Meal 2:
200g grilled chicken breast seasoned with chilli or herbs
Veg (usually spinach, lettuce, cucumber, green beans)
Extra virgin olive oil

3 hours later

Meal 3 (60 mins before the gym):
200g lean beef mince
30g cheese (usually cheddar)
Wholemeal bagel (made into a burger with the

beef mince and cheese)
Veg on the side

Meal 4 (immediately after training):
2 scoops of mint whey protein with water and 5g creatine
2 chocolate Rice Krispy squares or Coco Pops (with
unsweetened almond milk)

1-2 hours later

Meal 5:
Repeat meal 2 but add 250g of sweet potato
3 hours later

Meal 6:
200g of sirloin steak
Vegetables
Handful of nuts (usually cashews) or a shot of olive oil

Supplements:
3g of fish oils
500mg of curcumin
5000 IU of vitamin D3

(As I've stated previously, as the diet progresses, the carbs
from those meals will eventually end up being lower and
lower).

**Nutrient timing - "What and when should I eat before and
after the gym?"**

Let's discuss the topic of nutrient timing. Nutrient timing
is simply what and when you eat. More specifically, though,
it's often related to what someone eats before, during, and

after their resistance training session in the gym. This is something I am frequently asked about.

Please remember that that nutrient timing is way down the pecking order of importance compared to meeting your daily calorie needs, your protein needs, and simply choosing foods you get on well with. Nutrient timing can be added in once those other factors are being adhered to consistently. Having said that, it's worth considering, because while some foods around training can make you feel great, others can ruin your whole session. I learnt that the hard way once. I found that having fried eggs was not a great choice for me before training, as it didn't take long to throw them back up into the gym's bin. Now I steer clear of them before training.

I'm not going to be able to provide black and white guidelines here, as it's so unique to you as an individual and your goal. However, I will write this with someone in mind that wants to lose some flab, while potentially building some muscle; nothing too extreme, but they certainly don't want to end up looking skinny.

The purposes of correct nutrient timing are:

1. To ensure you have adequate energy to perform at your best
2. To increase the chance of muscle building
3. To reduce the risk of any muscle breakdown

The **protein** you eat around training plays a crucial role. It is responsible for ensuring that you increase muscle protein synthesis (MPS) during training. MPS is simply the process of building new proteins; or in other words, more muscle. This is an important aspect of creating a physique that looks strong and muscular.

Fats will slow down digestion. This is ideal, as it will allow your meal to provide a steadier release of energy, which is what you what, as you might not eat again for another 2-3 hours.

The benefits of consuming **carbs** around training are twofold. Firstly, they will provide you with some energy for the training session. Secondly, they will help to reduce muscle breakdown through the release of insulin (Chow, 2006). For those of you who take part in endurance training that lasts over 90 mins, then those carbs will help to replenish your glycogen levels (Aragon, 2008). Glycogen is simply what stored carbs are called, and they can be stored in the liver and muscle itself. This won't be so much of benefit for weight training sessions, as it's highly unlikely you will ever be that depleted (Aragon, 2008), unless you've chosen a very low carb approach. I'll use this section to add that I believe that if you want optimal results from your training and dieting, you are best to place as many of your daily carbs as you can around training as possible. Around training, your body will use those carbs far better than at any time of the day; and from my experience, this often leads to people getting better results.

Now that we have covered why each macronutrient is beneficial, we can look at some practical applications for what and when to eat around training.

Pre-workout

If you're eating a whole food meal before training, then I suggest eating it 60-90 minutes prior. You'll need to allow time for the food to digest before you begin training. This will vary from person to person, and for different foods, so play around with this and find what works for you. If you don't have time to eat that soon before training – for example, if you train in the morning after literally getting out of bed – then a liquid meal is a better choice, 30 minutes before training. For protein, 25g-50g is plenty to do its job. I find that leaner choices tend to work well for me and my clients. That means that you should be reaching for chicken breast, turkey breast, or a white fish for your pre-workout meal. The reason for this is that the overall fat you get from the meal will be lower and it will digest faster. If using a liquid meal, then a whey protein powder is ideal.

As I said above, fats are used to simply slow down the digestion a little bit. This is to prevent your blood sugars rising quickly and then crashing during training, which can make people feel crappy and may hinder performance. You don't want too much fat though, or your meal will sit in your gut for too long, and you run the risk of having to train while feeling bloated. I tend to have clients have between 5 and 15g of fat pre-workout. Having said that, if a client prefers a bit more or less than that, it isn't a problem. For myself, I usually have 10g. In terms of good sources of fat, I don't think it overly matters. My go-to sources will be extra virgin olive oil or a small portion of nuts.

You'll be best choosing carbs that will provide you with a slower release of energy, such as porridge oats, rice, and sweet potato. As with protein, 25-50g is usually plenty for pre-workout carbs. I know that for myself, if I eat too many carbs before training, they tend to make me feel tired. In fact, sometimes I'll even train with a relatively small amount of carbs – just 20g. Again, this will not only be personal preference, but also you must consider how many grams of carbs you have for the entire day. If you have chosen a lower carb diet, say 70g, then it makes no sense to eat 50g before training.

Your pre-workout will be dictated ultimately by foods you

digest well, and how long prior to training you can eat.

My (typical) pre-workout meal:
- 200g of grilled chicken breast
- 50g sweet potato
- 10g of extra virgin olive oil (I do it as a "shot" for ease and hardcore-ness)

This provides me with 50g protein, 50g carbs, and 5g fat. This is 490 calories, and I'll eat this roughly 60 minutes before I begin.

Intra-workout drinks

Intra-workout drinks are consumed while training. I don't tend to have clients use anything during training apart from water and electrolytes. The only time I have clients consume a liquid "meal" during their training while dieting is when they train early in the morning and they live close to the gym. I've already said that if you train early in the morning, then your pre-workout meal could be a liquid blend. Well, your other option is to have a carb and protein drink while you train. This really comes down to your personal preference, and I don't see either option being much different.

The only thing I'd suggest is that you don't have any fats added to the drink. You're already training, and therefore the concern for slowing down the energy release isn't there. Therefore, you would simply have carbs and protein. Whole protein sources like PeptoPro, which is basically a "predigested" protein source that you can drink, are a good option. The only downside is that it's also fairly expensive. Your other (and far cheaper) option is to purchase an essential amino acid powder and add 5-10g to your water. If you choose this option, then you will have to ensure that you have more protein immediately after training.

Currently, the best carb source for consuming while training is called highly-branched cyclin dextrin, or HBCD for short. The benefit of this powdered carb over more common choices like dextrose or glucose, which you'll find in sports drinks, is that it is digested far, far better. This means that most people won't experience any stomach upset or bloating while drinking it during training. That doesn't mean that more common sports drinks won't work.

Post-workout

The post-workout meal is the one that there is the most confusion about. This is most likely a byproduct of clever marketing from supplement companies that want you to use their products. Firstly, you don't have to eat something the very second you finish your last rep in the weights room! However, I do believe consuming something within an hour should be your priority. This gives most people enough time to head home and have a normal meal, should that be your preference. If you are training early in the morning and may have only had one small pre-workout shake, this, I feel, makes the post-workout meal even more important.

Having said that, I prefer to consume a whey protein shake after training. This is usually more because my appetite is suppressed after training due to the intensity. Again, similar to the pre-workout meal, 25-50g will be sufficient for most.

For a long time, most people recommended to keep fat as low as possible with the post-workout meal because of the fact it slows downs digestion, and therefore will slow down the release of glucose. The theory was that after training, you would need to deliver nutrients (protein and carbs) to your muscles as fast as possible, and fat would hinder this. Research into the subject doesn't seem to support any of these concerns (Aragon, 2008). Regardless, I still do a low-fat post-workout meal because I don't like how the fat makes me feel after training. After training, most of your blood is still sitting in the muscles you have just worked, and I don't feel that is the best time for digestion. Therefore, I just ensure I don't add any extra fat to my meal, and just consume what comes naturally from my carbs. If I was going to recommend having fat in this meal, I wouldn't go over 10g. This is something you can, of course, play around with.

Lastly, there are the carbs. This is a time I actually favour having more carbs than the rest of the day. This will naturally be limited by your total carb allowance for the day, but it isn't uncommon to have clients on 75-100g after training. Remember, we want to cause an insulin release for its ability to reverse the muscle breakdown caused by your training. Therefore, I favour high glycemic index (high GI) carbs that cause the largest rise in blood sugars after training. Good choices here are kids' cereals like Coco Pops, sweets and jelly beans, and low-fat pancakes with syrup. My personal go-to is Rice Krispy Squares. They have ~25g of carbs per bar and are fairly low in fat. They also taste nice and are easy to pack into a training bag.

You're best off consuming protein and carbs together, because the combination of the two will prevent muscle breakdown and fill your muscles back up better than they would do separately (Biolo et al., 1999; Zawadzki, Yaspelkis and Ivy, 1992).

My (typical) post-workout meal:
75g of whey protein isolate
Water
4 x Rice Krispy Squares

In summary:

Here is how I recommend you place your macronutrients in your diet before, during, and after training, as well as how much of each you'll need.

Meal	Protein	Fat	Carbs	Timing
Pre w/o	25-50g	5-10g	25-50g	30-90 mins
Intra w/o	25g	0g	25-50g	During
Post w/o	25-50g	low-10g based on preference	25-100g	0-60 mins

Water intake – "How much water do I need?"

Water intake is certainly an area that many beginners struggle with. I'll often have a client return their questionnaire and it will tell me that they often only manage a single glass of water each day, at best. I'm sure I don't need to go into detail about why you need to drink an adequate amount of water to ensure you are hydrated. Being dehydrated just 2% can affect your performance in the gym (Murray, 2007). Mild dehydration can also cause issues with mood, as well as problems with concentration, alertness, and short-term memory (Popkin, D'Anci and Rosenberg, 2010). This is not good if you are trying to run a successful business and need to be on the ball. Then, of course, if you end up too dehydrated, it can kill you.

So how much do you need? Well, to quote Lyle McDonald[12] , he states that "…a good rule of thumb is five clear urinations per day, and two of those should come after your workout"

12   Lyle is a very well-respected physiologist and nutritionist who does a great job of taking complicated exercise and fitness science and making is readily readable to the average person.

(McDonald, 2008). Ah, so this must be why men all look down when they are at the urinals. The key to this tip is going to be trial and error. So, for example, you might start with 4 glasses per day and see if you hit that "clear urination" quota. If you don't? Add a glass of water and repeat until you do. Simple. This actually makes a lot more sense than setting water intake strictly by bodyweight as some coaches will do, because some of you will sweat more than others, have more muscle than others, and some of you will live in warmer climates than the lovely English weather I'm accustomed to. I'd also note that you will want to gradually increase your water intake slowly over several days. If you go from one glass per day straight to six you will not only be running to the toilet pretty much nonstop, it can also be downright detrimental, as you'll suddenly dilute the level of sodium (salt) in the blood and this can cause some issues such as water retention, albeit only until the body readjusts.

One thing I can say is that most simply do not drink enough. It's not uncommon to get a food diary, to see that a client only drinks a glass of water per day. I'm certain that most of you reading this will benefit from increasing your water intake. Something to consider is that it isn't only water that will hydrate you. Tea, coffee, juices, milk, and even diet beverages will hydrate you (Grandjean et al., 2000). Keep that in mind. For most people, plain water isn't easy to consume, so you might consider flavouring it with sugar-free squash or fruits to make it easier to drink. This, like most things contained within this book, is just a new habit that you must stick at until it becomes something you don't have to think about doing. Until that time comes, it doesn't hurt to set alarms to remind you, and aim to have a bottle of water close to you at all times.

For those who do like black and white numbers, the NHS

still recommends 1.2L or 6-8 glasses per day (nhs.uk, 2017). To me, this seems very low, especially if you are doing resistance training and cardio. Having said that, this might be a good start for many of you to get to, and then see if you feel you need more.

Fibre – "Do I really have to eat my greens?"

The answer that question above is yes, yes you do. Well, you need some, of course, as you'll also get some fibre from the fruits and the other carbs in your diet.

According to the NHS' website, "Fibre is an important part of a healthy balanced diet. It can help prevent heart disease, diabetes, weight gain, and some cancers, and can also improve digestive health" (nhs.uk, 2015). There you go, it's good for you. I'll assume this isn't new information to any of you, but it's always worth reminding people of. A high-fibre diet can also help you poo. Constipation is something that, over the years, many of my clients have suffered with, and then improved once they have increased the fibre in their diets.

There are several reasons why a high-fibre diet helps with weight loss. The first is that it promotes fullness after a meal. It's very satiating. The good thing about fibrous foods is that they tend not to be very dense in calories, and therefore you can eat a substantial amount of them without using up your calorie allowance. This is especially true with greens like spinach, broccoli and kale, which I actually don't personally track or have my clients track.

Let's compare getting 20g of fibre from broccoli versus porridge oats. To get 20g of fibre from oats you would have to eat 180g and that would provide you with 700 calories. Now, to get 20g of fibre from broccoli you would need to eat 770g of broccoli and that gives you just 260 calories. I know what you're thinking: who the hell is going to eat nearly a kilo of broccoli per day? The answer to that is probably no one, barring some very extreme bodybuilders, perhaps. Of course, you will get your fibre from a mix of sources, but my point is still valid. You can get a fair amount of fibre from foods like green vegetables without using up too many precious calories. On a diet, when calories are limited, this is gold! When I was dieting for my competition and things got really rough, I would eat things like cucumber to fill me up (well try!) in between meals. Chances are you won't experience hunger like I did, but still, keep that in mind.

Fibre also slows down the rate at which food is digested and leaves the stomach, reduces the amount of nutrients the body actually uses, and keeps your blood sugar under control better. This is all extremely helpful for someone looking to lose weight while not feeling the negative effects of doing so, i.e. hunger. Of course, you'll still feel hungry at some point, but knowing these things and actually using them will make things slightly easier. These little wins add up if you implement them.

So how much do you need? The NHS recommends that try to eat at least 30g per day (nhs.uk, 2015). They also state that, on average, most people in the UK only eat around 18g. Not surprising, given what the average person in the UK typically eats. For those of you eating 3-5 meals per day, then you are looking at getting around 6-10g per meal. To put that into perspective, 6-10g of fibre in a single meal could be covered by:

- 50-100g of oats
- 200-300g of sweet potato
- 1-2 large apples
- 2-3 medium bananas

As you can see, you actually have to eat a fair amount of carbs to get those numbers; which is why, as I stated earlier, you'll be better off adding some form of fibrous vegetables to every meal from sources such as:

- Brussel sprouts
- Broccoli
- Spinach
- Kale
- Green beans
- Artichoke

To finish, I'd say I wouldn't stress out about hitting the targets. For many of you, simply adding in several servings of fruit, grains, and vegetables each day will provide you with all the fibre you'll need, and importantly, more than you are probably currently getting. If you pop your foods into an app, like I've suggested, you'll be able to see how much you are eating on a daily basis and make adjustments if needed.

Ending your diet – "How do I stop myself from regaining the weight I've lost?"

This could perhaps be the most important part of this entire book. Most of those who do manage to lose weight will find that keeping the weight off once they stop dieting can be extremely difficult. I doubt that surprises you one bit. If everyone who lost weight managed to maintain it, then the statistics on obesity would be vastly different! Many will actually go on to regain even more weight than they initially lost. Sadly, I've seen this happen many times.

One study, which analysed data from almost 300,000 people living in the UK over a ten-year period, concluded that "The probability of attaining normal weight or maintaining weight loss is low" (Fildes et al., 2015). Successful weight loss maintenance (which is defined as losing 10% or more of your body weight for more than a year) accounts for just 20% of dieters (Wing and Phelan, 2005). Those statistics fall lower and lower once you get past one year, as you can imagine. At the end of the day, weight loss should be a lifelong goal. I could provide plenty more stats like the ones above, but do you really need them? Just look around you, and you'll see that when it comes to losing weight and keeping it off, things aren't looking great.

Don't let that put you off, as you have a secret weapon: this book. This whole book has been written to make losing weight and maintaining that weight loss easier (which hopefully, by now you'll believe it will be). I believe if you lose weight the right way, and by that, I mean with a plan that doesn't make you want to kill yourself, then you will be far likelier to sustain your new lifestyle after the diet has ended. In that last sentence alone, I've let slip the key to getting this fitness thing right long-term. Using this book, you're going to create a new lifestyle, not a diet plan. The difference being that one is something we realise is done long-term, while the other (the diet) is something that is usually done in the short term. The issue with the latter is that once you end the so-called diet and go back to your old ways, you rapidly gain weight.

Unfortunately, this isn't the only thing we need to discuss when it comes maintaining your weight after you have achieved your goal. There is much more to consider. During a dieting phase where you are in a calorie deficit, the body gets pulled away from where it is most comfortable. The body doesn't overly like change, and so if you have been a certain weight for a long time, believe me, it isn't going to take too kindly to you trying to mess with that. In order to maintain your current weight, many hormones adapt which make it harder to continue. Over time, you become much hungrier than usual, and meals begin to feel less filling. There is also the issue of being low on energy, which causes you to move far less. Where you might once have walked the stairs, you are now taking the lift, and this means that on a daily basis, you are burning fewer calories. This can slow down your progress and make things more frustrating. Lastly, your metabolic rate will be lower, meaning you will need fewer calories per day to maintain your weight. All of this means that stopping the diet is difficult.

The issues of ongoing hunger and not feeling full

One of the main problems most have is that the end of a diet feels like the light at the end of the tunnel. It's something that you'll focus on to stay motivated. The hunger and the lack of feeling full are much more tolerable when you're close to achieving your goal and you're seeing some great changes in the mirror, while also feeling the health benefits. Problems tend to arise when you stop dieting. Most would expect all these feelings to go away, but they don't – well, not right away. For many, this comes as a shock. The reality now is that you must accept that you're not actually dieting anymore (and therefore don't have the same motivation), yet you will continue to feel like you are for several weeks. This is because dieting messes with hormones like Ghrelin (the hunger hormone) and leptin (the fullness hormone).

Often the real issue at this point is that you now have less self-control and motivation, because in your mind the diet is over. This makes it very difficult to not continue eating, to satisfy the hunger, even when you may have met your calorie requirements for the day. Regaining fat at this point in time is so easy to do, and this is one of the reasons that maintaining your new weight can be difficult.

Something I urge you all to do is not over-diet to the point where it's a daily struggle to stay motivated. Ending a diet at this point is risky. Bear in mind what I've already said: you are going to feel like you're dieting for a few more weeks. It can be hard to push yourself for those extra weeks; I know because I have experienced it. In 2015, when I did my bodybuilding competition, I dieted for 26 weeks. I gave literally everything to get to that show day, and getting 2nd place felt amazing. The problem was that I'd qualified for the British finals just two weeks later. The issue was that I'd prepared myself for 26 weeks of dieting. I wasn't mentally ready for two extra weeks, and I'll admit, I didn't think I'd make it! It was carnage going back to that diet, on top of three hours of training, six days per week.

A safer option, albeit somewhat slower, would be to diet and stop a few weeks short of it being horrible. That way, you won't feel like crap, and you'll find that you have a little more motivation to stay strong once it's over. So instead of dieting for 16 weeks, you may stop at 12. Sure, you won't lose as much, but let's remember that losing 6kg and keeping 6kg off beats losing 8kg and regaining 8kg, which is very common. Remember, if you maintain your weight and keep yourself sane, there is no reason why you can't then do another dieting phase. I often do this with my own clients – very successfully, I might add. If someone has, for example, 10kg to lose, we might diet for six weeks to lose half of that weight, and then take a two- to four-week diet break, which gives the body and the mind a chance to recover. After taking that break, we will go back to dieting to lose the last 5kg. It's a much more effective strategy, believe me.

You don't need as much food after your diet ends

Unfortunately, your new trim, lean, healthier body doesn't need as many calories to maintain itself as you would have been eating prior to losing the weight. Calorie needs are based on your weight, as you have already seen from the calculations I've provided, and you are now lighter than you were before, unless you've built a lot of muscle at the same time to counter that fat loss. That is rare, but does happen, as I've proved already using my own clients as examples. You'll also have a slightly reduced metabolic rate as well, due to being on low calories, and most likely, lower carbs. This is why you simply can't just stop dieting and return to your old habits.

Here's a practical example of what I mean:

A guy who is active most days will need roughly 33 calories (although this can vary, 33 is a great starting point) per kilo of body weight to maintain his weight. If we take a 100kg male who then loses 15kg to end up at a weight of 85kg.

At his original weight of 100kg he would need ~3300 calories to be at maintenance.

At 85kg he only needs ~2805 calories for maintenance.

To account for the reduced metabolic rate caused by dieting, I use Lyle McDonald's recommendation of using 90% (McDonald, 2008) of this predicted amount and this leaves our guy requiring 2525 calorie per day.

Therefore, losing that 15kg has resulted in a massive reduction of 775 fewer calories per day than he needed before starting his diet.

If this guy does what most do after a diet and just returns to his old ways and eats at his maintenance of 3300 calories, or worse, more, those extra 775 calories each would be enough to gain 0.6kg a week; maybe more.

I would say this is me playing it pretty safe with the maths because what we can't really account for is how sensitive his body is to store fat after a diet. It's also very likely that he'll binge and gain even more weight than I've predicted. Basically, remember that it's very easy to regain fat once you stop dieting if you're not extremely careful. Hopefully, I've explained that well enough for you to understand why it's important to not see the end of your diet as the end of your new lifestyle. No wonder so many people regain the weight back so fast. This is where the term "yo-yo dieting" comes from. You lose weight, regain it, and then retry. Well, not anymore. Not under my watch!

The question is, then, what do you do? Well, this is actually not that difficult – if you're prepared to carry on being accountable for the foods and drinks you consume for just a little longer. If this can be done, then you will have a much greater chance of maintaining your new weight.

Your goal is to get your calorie intake back to maintenance levels as quickly as possible so that your body can begin to recover from the diet. I recommend following the guidelines from Lyle McDonald's article *The Transition Phase Between Dieting and Gaining* (McDonald, 2008), and putting your calories to 31-35 calories per kilo of current weight minus 10%. As Lyle states, "There is an adaptive decrease in energy expenditure that occurs during dieting that makes the estimated maintenance too high". In other words, let's be careful.

For some of you, one benefit of this approach is that it will also ease any worries that you will gain fat once you start to eat more. This is very common, and I totally understand it. After all the hard work you've put in, you don't want to screw it up! Follow my recommendations, and you'll be fine. I've yet to see one client gain a load of fat when they stick to the plan.

Just to be on the safe side, let's do another example:

So, if you ended your diet at 80kg you would go back to:

1. 80 x 31-35 = 2480 - 2800 calories per day
2. 2480 - 2800 x 0.9 = 2232 - 2520 calories per day

Your new diet plan would require between 2232 and 2520 calories per day.

You would then follow this new diet plan over the next 7-14 days, and observe your weight, measurements, and how you look in the mirror to determine if it was the right amount. If, after that period, your weight hasn't drastically increased (remember that it will initially go up a few kilos due to eating more food, and more carbs and water being stored in the muscle), you can increase the calories by 5-10% and then repeat the process. Of course, if you have overestimated the calories needed, simply reduce them by 5-10% and reassess.

After repeating that process a few times, you'll soon find the number of calories needed to maintain your weight. At this point, it would be a good idea to stay there for several weeks, even up to 12, to ensure you fully recover. Once your calories have been at maintenance long enough so that your body is happy with your new level of body fat, you could consider dieting again, if it's needed. Signs that your body has recovered are things such as:

- Reduced hunger
- Less cravings
- Increased energy
- The feeling of fullness after meals
- Libido is good
- Performance in the gym is increasing and
  you are getting stronger

In order to increase your calories, you are going to need to decide where these calories are going to come from (protein, fats, or carbs), and so I recommend the following:

Protein: I would keep the protein constant for the time being, as it will certainly help to keep your hunger at bay. It won't need to be increased, though.

Carbs: Carbs will definitely need to be higher, especially for those of you who ended up with them low by the end of the diet. By the end of my diet, I was down to just 50g per day. That lasted roughly eight weeks, if I recall correctly. Carb levels this low will affect your thyroid and therefore cause a slowdown in your metabolism. To quote Lyle McDonald's article again, he states that "One critical aspect is that carbohydrate intake should be brought to 120-150 grams per day as a minimum (1-1.5 g/lb would be a good rough estimate for all but the most non-behemoth men)". This is the equivalent of 2.2-3.3g of carbs per kilo of body weight.

Of course, you can go higher, but this seems to be the minimum needed for a full thyroid recovery after a diet.

Fats: With protein and carbs already being set, you can simply get the rest of the calories from some good fats.

Example:
Using our 80kg man as the example again, let's assume he's fairly active and has opted for the higher end of the scale, and is eating 2500 calories per day.

1. Protein is 210g per day = 840 calories
2. Carbs are 260g per day = 1040 calories
3. This leaves him with 620 calories for fat. 620/9 = 68.9 (round fat to 70g)

His new diet looks like this:
Calories = 2500
Protein = 210g
Carbs = 260g
Fat = 70g

Changes to training post-diet

It might not seem too obvious, but after you stop dieting, you will also have to consider how you'll go about reducing any aerobic cardio training you were doing in order to maintain a calorie deficit. If, by the end of your diet, you were doing five to six sessions of 30-60 minutes, then you're definitely not going to want to continue doing this. Remember that your goal post-diet is physical recovery. One benefit of reducing your cardio is that you'll begin to recover better from your training, and this allows you to make more progress. In more concrete terms, this means that you will gain more muscle and strength.

Because you'll have already added some extra calories back into your diet, you will have to be careful with any reductions you make to your cardio. Reducing how many calories you burn per day affects the energy balance, no different to adding in more calories. This is something to be cautious about. If you add in 200 calories per day AND reduce calorie burning by 200 calories per day, you get a net change of 400. If you don't consider this, you could easily end up with an energy balance over your maintenance.

For this reason, I will rarely just remove a client's cardio altogether, instead choosing to remove around 50% of it. If they were completing five sessions of 60 mins, they might drop to 5 sessions of 30 minutes. Again, the key here is to observe how this affects your body over a few weeks. Like with food increases, if everything is okay, I will remove another 50% of the week's cardio. At this point, instead of doing five sessions of 15 minutes, a total of 75 minutes, I will be more likely to do 3 sessions of 25 minutes, simply so they don't have to go to the gym as often. Once cardio is this low, you could then drop it to three sessions of 20 mins per week. This way, you can reap the benefits associated with aerobic work without making it needlessly difficult to recover from weight sessions. Due to more food, carbs especially, you will begin to feel a lot more productive after the diet is over.

Weight training could also be reduced slightly, if needed, for a week or two. Again, this is to allow for some extra recovery. You could simply reduce how many times a week you have been doing weight training by one day. If you've been doing four weight training sessions, you would reduce that to three. I don't think this is the most crucial thing to worry about. Adding in more food and doing less aerobic sessions will make a huge difference to how you feel. Reducing weight training sessions would be a good idea if you have any niggling injuries. If you feel okay, though, I would recommend trying to maintain your weight training where it is, for the time being.

Some key points –

1. Put calories back to 31-35 cals/kg/bw minus 10%
2. Reduce cardio by 50%
3. If needed, reduce training days by one day for a week or two.
4. Follow this new plan for two to three weeks and reassess. If body weight is stable, add 5-10% more calories and decrease cardio a further 50%
5. Repeat this until weight starts to rise slightly so you know where to stop.

Refeeds – "When can I have a cheat meal?"

One of the first questions that I'll probably receive from a new client is, "When will I get a cheat meal?". Strangely, it's not uncommon to be asked this before the diet has even begun! To be honest, I guess I really don't blame them. Knowing when you might get a curry, some pizza, or a glass of wine gives you something to look forward to. As much as I'd recommend choosing to eat whole, unprocessed foods the majority of the time, there are reasons why having something you enjoy from time to time can be beneficial.

The psychological benefits

The obvious benefits of having an "off-plan" meal is that it will give you a much-needed psychological boost.

It's unrealistic to assume that you'll be able to diet 8, 10, 12 weeks without wanting something that you're craving. In fact, I think trying to do so really reduces your chances of long-term success. At the point when all you can think about is food, hunger is high, and cravings are beginning to creep in, it's very helpful to know that you are going to have a meal you like soon. It's a much better idea than thinking, "I promised myself I'd stay strict for at least six weeks".

Personally, I believe that eating these sorts of foods from time to time also helps to build a good relationship with food. Too many people struggle to include the foods they really like within their diet in a sensible, controlled manner. They will instead binge on these foods, and then they feel guilty. It's also terribly unhealthy, as well. Understanding that it's just fine to eat something that you would normally believe is "bad" for weight loss and overall health is very powerful. No one ever got fat and unhealthy from a single day of eating a little junk food or having a few glasses of wine. This means that dieting can be flexible, as long as you can stay in control.

Control is the key to making this work for you. If you want to enjoy the occasional indulgence, eat a meal of your choosing at some point during the day. Before that meal, and as soon as you finish that meal, you continue eating your regular foods, and carry on with the plan as intended. There is no domino effect, where that one meal turns into a binge; or worse, a binge lasting several days.

The physiological benefits

What many people won't know is that eating foods that provide more calories and more sugar can actually help with fat loss. Yep, you read that right: for optimal fat loss, it would be sensible to include small periods of deliberate "over-feeding", and this is referred to as a "refeed". As I've already mentioned, when you begin dieting to lose body fat, the body reacts by slowing down your metabolism in an effort to maintain a stable body weight. We also know that changes in certain hormones mean that you'll feel hungrier than usual, while beginning to feel less "full" from your meals. Also note that free testosterone levels can begin to drop, meaning muscle loss and a lowered libido. As you can imagine, this is all less than ideal when it comes to changing your body and improving your health!

This is where the "refeeds" come in. The extra calories (and carbs, which will raise insulin) can help to reverse all of the negative factors associated with dieting. This effect will be brief, as you're going to have to return back to your diet straight away. With my clients, I personally use a method of refeeding called "skiploading". Skiploading was developed by Ken "Skip" Hill, a very well-known bodybuilding coach and someone who I'm very fortunate to call my mentor (he only chose five people from a lot of applicants!). Skiploading is a high-calorie day, usually done on a Saturday or Sunday, where a person would eat highly processed junk foods high in sugar (and sometimes fat, depending on the person). Skip has built his whole career and reputation on getting bodybuilders to appear "skinless" (as he often says), even with weekly junk food binges.

Too good to be true? Hell, no! To put it into perspective, I ended my competition diet on roughly 1750 calories a day. However, one Sunday, I tracked my skipload foods to find that I had in fact eaten 15,000 calories that day – in a ten-hour period, in fact (more on that in a minute). My go-to foods were:

- Cereals like Coco Pops with low fat milk or almond milk
- Pancakes covered in syrup
- Rice Krispy Squares
- Jam on toast (white bread, of course)
- Pizza
- Cookies

But that doesn't mean you couldn't have foods like:

- Burger and chips
- Sushi with rice

I think I've made my point. Imagine that your metabolism is a fire, and over the course of several weeks of dieting, the fire begins to go out. Well, Skip describes a skipload as "pouring gas [petrol to you and me] on a fire". The gas helps to reignite the fire to burn hotter. This is what taking extra calories and sugar does to your metabolism.

A study has actually tested this theory (Davoodi et al., 2014). It took overweight women and compared the difference in weight loss between a classic calorie restriction (CR) diet and a calorie shifting diet (CSD), which is another of saying they had days where the calories were higher. The CSD group did 11 days of normal dieting followed by 3 days where they could self-select their foods. This cycle of eating behaviour was repeated for six weeks. They then had a four-week follow-up period.

The results were not surprising to someone like myself, who has seen bodybuilders diet like this for many years, but the average person would probably be rather shocked. The group who did the CSD diet lost more weight, had better adherence, their metabolisms hadn't changed, and their feelings of hunger and fullness were improved after four weeks. The researchers concluded that not only did they lose more fat during the diet, the diet affected them less after. This reduced their chances of regaining the weight.

I've been using refeed days for a few years now, and can safely say that I don't think I'll ever diet any other way. I'm sure my clients agree.

Cheat meals

I'd like to briefly mention cheat meals. They are often seen as the same thing as a refeed to some people, but not me. Personally, I've never liked calling them "cheat meals", because the term "cheating" is so very negative. It implies that you've done something wrong, and I don't want my clients to see certain foods as bad. Most of my clients already have a poor relationship with food when they come to me, and I do not want to exacerbate this.

Apart from that, a cheat meal serves the same purpose as a refeed. However, I don't believe that a single meal will provide enough calories to truly make your body think, "Ah, all is okay! Food is available". In my opinion, a single cheat meal only provides psychological benefits, and therefore will not provide the same physiological benefits that a refeed day will. This makes cheat meals useless for ensuring that you get continued progress over the weeks.

I, therefore, prefer skiploading, as the skipload provides more and more calories over the weeks as you get further into a diet, and things get even harder.

The "how-to"

It's not going to be easy to give very specify instructions on how to do a skipload correctly, as there are so many variables, but I will try to provide you with enough information so that you can give it a try for yourself.

You won't need to refeed for several weeks, as your body does take time to be affected and to go into "starvation mode". Also, from experience, I'll add that it often takes my clients three to four weeks, at least, to really become accustomed to their new lifestyle. It takes time to form new habits, and get into the swing of things. Therefore, you will want to hold off from doing a refeed while you discover whether the diet plan you've set up is working for you.

With all of this in mind, I recommend waiting until you have got at least six weeks of <u>successful</u> dieting under your belt before you even consider it. You'll know when you are ready to do one because you will have lost several kilos, and you're beginning to see things slow down. Your energy will also begin to feel drained, and cravings will become almost impossible to ignore. If you're feeling like this, then it's time to eat.

Skiploads are done for a specific period of time. During this block of free time, you can eat almost freely (much like the study I discussed), and that block of free time can last anywhere from two hours to a full day, depending on the individual. I recommend that you all begin with just two hours. That is enough time to eat some foods that you like and have that mental break from dieting. For almost everyone, two hours is not going to ruin any of your efforts, and chances are high that you would need more time in the following week.

Once you've completed your allotted time, then you simply return to your normal diet for the rest of the day. Over the next seven days, you can then evaluate how that extra food has affected your weight. You <u>will</u> gain some weight because of the extra carbs and water that will be stored in the muscle as *glycogen*, and this will make you heavier. Think of your muscles as a sponge, which becomes heavier when submerged in water. I'll routinely gain around 6-7kg on a Sunday refeed when I'm dieting, just to put it into perspective. Over the course of the following week, you will sweat some water off and use some of those stored carbs for training, and your weight will fall again. You are looking to see whether your weight falls below what your previous *lowest weight* was.

If you do get a good weight drop of 0.5-1kg, then you can add an another hour the following week. If your weight drop doesn't drop below the previous low, and you are left where you were before you did you refeed, then this is usually a sign that the diet (or your activity) in the week needs to be adjusted to get you back into a calorie deficit. Do this as shown earlier in this book.

Key points:

- As you diet, your metabolism will slow down.
- Over time, you will crave foods you miss and enjoy, and the diet will feel much harder.
- A high carb/calorie refeed can aid fat loss by boosting metabolism and motivation.
- Some do a one-off meal known as a "cheat meal", while others may do refeeds for a specific amount of time. In bodybuilding, this is commonly called a "skipload", after coach Ken "Skip" Hill who made this style of diet popular by getting excellent results.
- High-carb junk foods like cereals and sweets work very well.
- These foods will make your weight rise initially due to extra carbs and water stored in the muscles.
- This extra weight should drop over the course of five to seven days, along with another 0.5-1kg.

- If your weight doesn't drop below your previous low, then you should adjust your normal diet plan (or activity) as shown earlier in the book.

Salt intake - "What about my blood pressure?"

Let's dive into the subject of salt, shall we? The salt we get from the foods we consume provides us with the mineral sodium. In this section, I may flip from talking about salt to sodium, so just remember that we get sodium from salt.

The main roles of sodium within the body are:

1. It controls water balance within the body and the cells. It, therefore, affects blood volume, as well. The body has ways to ensure that water in the body is tightly controlled. This is the way in which it affects your blood pressure (more on that in a mo).

2. Sodium is an electrolyte. Electrolytes carry the electrical current needed to keep nerves, organs, and muscles functioning correctly. Sodium is also needed for strong muscle contractions. At the gym, you may be able to notice if your sodium is too low, because you won't feel like your muscles "squeeze" very well.

Salt and your health

It's clear that we do need sodium. The problem is that, on average, adults in the UK consume too much salt, and this has been linked to causing high blood pressure (He and MacGregor, 2007). Having high blood pressure increases your chances of strokes, cardiovascular diseases, and kidney disease. Unfortunately, it can be easy to consume too much salt, because it's added to a lot of "ready-made" and processed foods, and it's highly likely that you are getting the majority of your nutrition from those foods. The question really is: how much salt should we be getting?

Evidence suggests that if you bring your salt intake down to the recommended intake of 6g per day, it will reduce your blood pressure (Ha, 2014). This should be a pretty easy fix once you begin choosing to eat more lean cuts of meat, fish, eggs, healthy fats, vegetables and fruit. To highlight that point, I'll use my own diet as an example. I eat six meals per day, on average. This therefore means that, on average, I can consume 1g of salt per meal.

A typical meal for me, looks something like this:

- 200g of chicken breast = 0.37g of salt
- 200g of sweet potato = 0.28g
- 10g of olive oil = 0.001g
- Total salt = 0.65g

That is a typical meal for me, which I will eat three times over the course of the day. The other three meals will come from protein shakes. Those meals also contain well under 1g of salt in them. The only meal that would go over my 1g allowance would be the one after training. That meal would contain closer to 2g of salt. I'm not overly concerned here. I train for 60-90 minutes and I tend to sweat a lot! That sweat will cause sodium loss, and that sodium will need to be replaced. My point is that if you choose "healthy" foods, this will instantly reduce your salt intake rather well.

I should acknowledge that some studies have shown that high sodium intake doesn't cause any increased health risks to people with normal blood pressure (Mente et al., 2016), which will describe many of you, I'm sure. One study concluded that "...these data suggest that lowering sodium intake is best targeted at populations with hypertension who consume high sodium diets" (Mente et al., 2016).

You also have to consider that salt is only one small factor in the equation. The most important factor for blood pressure is still your weight, with overweight people, of course, being likelier to have high blood pressure (Lelong et al., 2014). I'd be interested to see someone with high blood pressure maintain their high salt intake while losing body fat, to see if the lifestyle changes needed to accomplish this reduced their blood pressure. Your primary focus for optimal health should still be to lose weight. This alone will have a profound effect on your health.

It's worth noting that it can be unhealthy to go too low. As with excessive sodium intakes, low intakes are also associated with higher death rates (Graudal et al., 2014). Strangely, these studies gave an ideal "healthy" range of roughly 6g to 12g – double the actual current recommendations in the UK. It seems that the research is not yet entirely conclusive.

At this point in time, I would suggest you stick to the recommended 6g of salt per day. If you are using a food tracking app like I've suggested, then along with protein, fats, and carbs, it will also track sodium intake, making it fairly easy to be accountable for. Like I have shown with my food examples, switching to unprocessed, homemade meals will pretty much do the job. However, if you're someone who eats out frequently, you'll have to be careful, as you won't be able to account for the salt that's added to your food or used to cook with. It should also go without saying that everyone should probably be keeping an eye on their blood pressure a few times a week. A blood pressure monitor is cheap and extremely important if you value your health.

The sodium-potassium ratio

If you do have high blood pressure, it's also possible to lower it by increasing the amount of potassium in your diet. Your blood pressure is regulated by the amount of water you retain in the body, and this is controlled by the ratio of sodium to potassium. If your sodium intake is high, and is causing high blood pressure, you can get the same result by increasing your potassium intake. Foods such as these are great options:

- Avocado
- Spinach
- Sweet potato
- Coconut water
- Banana
- Yogurt
- Beans

The recommended intake of potassium is 3.5g. Again, use your food tracking app to ensure you're meeting those needs. If not, you can increase it using the foods listed above.

Recommended supplements – "What ones shall I use to lose weight faster?"

Before we get into this chapter, I want you to remember that supplements are meant to complement your diet and training regime, not to be used as a crutch. Remember, there are a lot of companies out there selling supplements that you will never need to use and, in many cases, don't even work anyway. Unless your idea of "losing a few pounds" is destroying your bank balance, I suggest you think carefully about which supplements you commit to using.

I'm not medically trained, and so I would recommend you

all head to your GP for blood tests if you really want a clear idea of what supplements would help you. That being said, there are several supplements that I believe every one of you reading this will benefit from taking.

Fish oils/Essential fatty acids

There is a good chance that many of you will be eating a far greater amount of omega-6 fatty acids (polyunsaturated fats) from foods such as vegetable oils, nuts, seeds and certain junk foods per day, than you are omega-3 fatty acids, found in foods like salmon or mackerel. In fact, the optimal ratio of omega 3 to 6 is 1:1, yet some studies (Simopoulos, 2002) have shown that in the western diet, it's more like 15:1-16.7:1 in favour of omega 6. In other words, we overeat omega-6 and under-eat omega-3. High amounts of omega-6 fatty acids and a high omega-6/omega-3 ratio can promote cardiovascular disease, cancer, and issues caused by inflammation such, as arthritis and diabetes. Unless you're eating plenty of oily fish every day, I recommend you get yourself a quality fish oil.

There is evidence that supplementing with omega-3 can reduce triglycerides (so much so, in fact, that you can be prescribed a pharmaceutical version by the doctor), protect those with heart disease, relieve joint pain, reduce depression, and reduce inflammation (which, in my opinion, makes fish oils worthwhile on their own). There are plenty more benefits, but that should sell it pretty well.

You can get the supplement in liquid form or in pills. I've tried the flavoured liquids, and they are bad at best, so I switched back to the pills. What you are looking for is a product that has a good concentration of EPA (eicosapentaenoic acid) and DHA (docosahexaenoic acid). Don't be fooled, many fish oil pills are marketed as being 1000mg, but within that 1000mg, you might only get 250mg of combined EPA and

DHA. I had a client once who got a real cheap brand that was so low in EPA/DHA that she needed 12 pills a day to get the correct amount. This is worrying, given that the "serving suggestion" was just *one to two pills daily.*

Speaking of recommended amounts, I can hear you asking, "How much do I need?". The American Heart Association recommends that, if you have coronary heart disease, you take 1,000 mg of EPA and DHA daily (Frank et al., 2017); but if someone needs to lower triglycerides, for example, they recommend 2000-4000mg each day (naturalproductsinsider. com, 2011). If you research a recommended dose, you'll be pushed to find something set in stone, currently. As a minimum, then, I'd recommend 1000mg of EPA/DHA daily, but personally suggest you go for 2000-3000mg per day. With the ones I'm currently using, that is only three to four pills. I usually split them into two doses a day: one in the morning with breakfast, and one with my last meal. If you have a specific condition or issue you're trying to combat with fish oils, then I would suggest either speaking to your doctor or doing some research online to see if you can find some better guidelines for your particular needs.

Finally, if you are a vegetarian or vegan, then you can get your essential fatty acids from flaxseed oil. Flax seed oil will provide you with alpha-linolenic acid (ALA), which the body can then convert to EPA/DHA. The problem is the conversion of ALA to DHA in the body has been shown to be awful, at just 0.1%, while ALA to EPA conversation is just 0.3% (Hussein et al., 2004). Your best option is to stick to the fish oils.

Vitamin D3

If you're reading this in the UK, then I probably won't need to convince you that you will most likely need to supplement with vitamin D3 to increase your levels in the body – we are hardly basking in glorious sunshine, are we? In the UK, it's been shown that more than half of adults don't get enough vitamin D during the winter and spring, and that 16% are severely deficient (Power and Hyppönen, 2007).

Vitamin D is a fat-soluble nutrient. It helps the body absorb and regulate calcium and phosphate, which, of course, helps us maintain strong bones and teeth, and helps with muscle contractions (something you'll need to get into better shape, of course). Other benefits include improvements in immune function, as well as a reduced risk of heart disease, diabetes, and colorectal cancer (Gorham et al., 2007). Vitamin D3 supplementation that puts your levels at an optimal level may also be beneficial for testosterone production (Pilz et al., 2010, Wehr et al., 2009) – something every ageing guy should be concerned about.

That's why you should consider adding it to your plan. You *may* get away no supplementation in the summer, if you're someone who likes to be in the sun. With all the scaremongering about skin cancer nowadays, it's likely that you may actually avoid getting some UVB rays, and therefore will need to supplement year-round. It's very hard to get some concrete numbers on this, but the Vitamin D Council states, "You don't need to tan or to burn your skin in order to get the vitamin D you need. Exposing your skin for a short time will make all the vitamin D your body can produce in one day. In fact, your body can produce 10,000 to 25,000IU of vitamin D in just a little under the time it takes for your skin to turn pink" (Vitamindcouncil.org, 2017). The issue is that this will vary from person to person depending on many factors, so you might just want to get some sun for 10-30 minutes, but certainly stop before you start to look like a lobster.

Bear in mind that I just stated that even a little direct sunlight can allow the body to produce thousands of IUs of vitamin D a day; yet interestingly, some organisations are still recommending daily intakes as low as 400IU per day. Some research studies and organisations have set a safe upper limit of 10,000 IU per day. The Vitamin D Council have a higher recommended dose of 5,000 IU per day (Cannell, 2013), and this is the amount I take myself.

I tend to start clients on 2,500 IU to begin with, but will have them get it tested. This is the best way to be sure. I had mine tested recently during one of my semiannual health "mots", and mine was actually a little low. This allowed me to address the situation by increasing my daily dose. The test you will give you your vitamin D [25(OH)D] levels. Several studies have concluded that "optimal vitamin D status was achieved when 25(OH)D3 was > 100 nmol/L" (Norman, 2008). You will be fine, however, if you have levels that range between 75 and 125 nmol/L.

Should a blood test come back with low levels of vitamin D, it's worth noting that taking 100 IU of vitamin D3 will raise blood levels by 2.5 nmol/L (Moyad, 2008). Let's imagine you get yours tested, and the doctor tells you that your vitamin D came back as low at 35 nmol/L. To get into range, you'll need to raise your blood levels by at least 40 nmol/L. Still with me?

So we get:
1. nmol needed to be in range/2.5 x 100
2. 40/2.5 x 100 = 1,600 IUs of vitamin D3 needed.

Vitamin D3 needs to be taken with the fats from a meal (or your fish oils), and, if desired, can conveniently be taken as *one single weekly dose*. I've found this to be great when

I'm busy and I'm very likely to forget. Once you reach the level you desire (found by retesting, of course), you would probably drop back to a lower dose and maintain; but again, I'd recommend speaking to your GP about this.

Vitamin K2

Vitamin K2 is something I've recently added myself, and have started recommending to my clients. I feel K2 is a good addition to the supplement regime for older guys due to its ability to prevent the calcification and stiffening of the arteries (Beulens et al., 2009, Geleijnse et al., 2004). This, of course, reduces your risk of cardiovascular disease, like heart attacks. It also plays an important role in bone health by improving bone mineral density. In other words, it'll reduce the risk of osteoporosis (Frank et al., 2017), which is another great benefit of ensuring you get adequate amounts. Vitamin K supplementation has also been shown to be a good tool for cancer therapy, where it could reduce the likelihood of liver cancer reoccurring (Kubota et al., 2012).

You can get this vitamin from food, but getting the ideal amount can be difficult and is fairly uncommon. Good examples of foods containing higher amounts of Vitamin K2 are:

- Veggies like kale, cabbage, broccoli, asparagus
- Egg yolk
- Butter
- Dairy
- Prunes
- Meats

You might want to ensure you get the right amount by using a supplement. Vitamin K2 will be named as menaquinones on the labels of supplements. There are actually different types of menaquinones that will be abbreviated as MK-4, 7, 8, or 9, and this changes the amount required. This is worth knowing when you go to purchase a particular brand.

- Vitamin K2 as MK-4 has a minimum effective dose of 1500mcg (Frank et al., 2017)
- Vitamin K2 as MK-7/8/9 has a minimum effective dose between 90 and 360mcg (Frank et al., 2017)

Vitamin K2 is a fat-soluble vitamin, which means you'll need to take it with a meal containing fats or with your fish oils. There is research that suggests that vitamin K2 works even better when combined with vitamin D3, because they will work synergistically (Kid, 2010). This is why, at the time of writing this, I am using (and recommending clients use the same) a supplement by Life Extension that contains vitamin D3 and vitamin K2 (as well as Iodine). It can be found at **www.lifeextensioneurope.co.uk**

Curcumin

Curcumin is the amazing ingredient that's extracted from the spice turmeric (which gives curry its yellow colour) and is getting a lot of attention nowadays, and rightly so. Curcumin is a very good anti-inflammatory (Chainani-Wu, 2003, Hanai et al., 2006), and boasts many other benefits, such as:

- Being a potent antioxidant (DiSilvestro et al., 2012)
- Decreasing depression (Lopresti et al., 2014)
- Aiding in pain relief (Agarwal et al., 2011)
- Reducing anxiety (Esmaily et al., 2015)

There are many more, and there are plenty of studies to bolster those claims, hence why it is something I recommend everyone should be taking.

The recommended dose for curcumin is 80-500mg (Frank et al., 2017). This is the dose needed if you have a product that has good bioavailability. The issue with curcumin is that absorption by the body can be poor, meaning that although you may be taking a good dose of the stuff, it might not actually be doing its job. Therefore, you have to get a product that has improved absorption by adding black pepper (piperine) to it, or one that states it's using a patented curcumin such as Meriva or BCM-95. I personally use the one from Life Extension, which provides me with 400mg of BCM-95 curcumin daily in just one pill. 400mg is the dose I have my clients take daily, and we have seen some great results in doing so, mostly coming from its ability to reduce inflammation and pain. This really does seem to help with past injuries and soreness.

Magnesium

Magnesium is a mineral that is one of several electrolytes needed by the body. Its role includes regulating blood pressure, maintaining normal nerve and muscle function, maintaining strong bones, and helping to keep your blood sugar levels stable. Although magnesium is fairly easy to get from a well-balanced diet, many people in the west are still deficient in this mineral because they will not choose to eat these foods. We all know that the average diet is pretty poor, so this isn't really a surprise. You could aim to get more magnesium from your diet by increasing the amount of the following foods in your diet:

- Dark leafy greens such as spinach, kale and chard
- Dark chocolate
- Nut and seeds such as pumpkin seeds, almonds and flax

- Oily fish such as mackerel, salmon and tuna
- Avocado
- Banana
- Yogurt

If you are someone who doesn't consistently consume these foods, then 400-500mg per day of a quality magnesium citrate (Frank et al., 2017) supplement will be a good option.

I recommend that my clients take it 30 minutes before going to bed, because magnesium is known to aid sleep in many people. In fact, one of my current clients literally can't stop going on about how well he is sleeping since he added the magnesium. He runs a very successful business and the stress of this has, over time, led to some insomnia. I would argue that it isn't just the magnesium helping, but the combination of the supplement, the better foods, the weight loss, and the exercise. However, he isn't the first client to be very pleased he started taking the supplement before bed, so give it a try and see how you get on.

Protein powders

I'm going to state straight away that protein shakes really aren't a necessity. By no means does anyone actually need to use them, no matter what most magazines and supplement companies will say. Having said that, let me explain why I still recommend getting yourself a decent protein powder. You can then make up your own minds.

Firstly, it's convenient. You can pop 1-2 scoops (~25-50g of protein) into a container, chuck it into your bag, and have it there for when you're too busy to grab some food, or if you are somewhere that doesn't have some quality protein for sale. For those of you who travel a lot, whether that's internationally or just up and down the country, taking some protein powder with you will make it easy to get a serving of quality protein quickly. Simply add water, shake and drink. Job done.

I also find them handy to have at the ready when I simply don't want to stop working. For example, they've been great while writing this book, because once I get into the flow of writing, I don't really want to stop to cook. Instead, I'll have a shake and some water next to me. The same will go for those of you who are too busy at times to stop for a proper meal.

They taste pretty good nowadays. I still remember my first protein shake from back when I was at school. I'd mix it up during my last class of the day in a bottle (no idea why I didn't have a shaker, as I'm sure they must have been around at that time. I'm not that old!). It was thick, gritty and it tasted like utter crap. Had it not been for the fact it was pink and said "strawberry" on the packaging, I seriously wouldn't have known what its intended flavour was. Thankfully, they are much nicer nowadays, my favourite being the "choc mint" one from www.theproteinworks.com. When you're dieting, many of you will often look forward to having something that tastes "sweet". When I diet, I like to use a chocolate protein shake mixed with water (but only a little to make it thicker) as "milk" to pour over my Coco Pops after training. It's a small treat to look forward to each day, especially when the rest of the day's food can be bland.

After training, a shake is often a much easier option to stomach than something like chicken or lean beef, which can be hard to digest, especially if you've worked hard. A shake is a good choice for those of you who might not be able to eat again for another couple of hours due to returning to work or having to commute home. Your best option here is to have a protein shake and then have a solid meal an hour or two after that.

I'll finish my reasons for at least having some protein powder on hand by saying that many of you will struggle to meet your daily protein needs in the beginning. This is probably one of the first "complaints" (I use that term loosely, as it's better to be full than hungry) that I get from new clients. If you are struggling to eat enough meat, fish and dairy to meet your protein requirements, then using a couple of protein shakes will be a lot bloody easier. A nice shake in a flavour you enjoy will always go down faster and easier than 200-250g of meat when you are feeling full up. Believe me. I tend to recommend clients have no more than three shakes per day, which, for many, will be half of their meals. If you are only eating three meals a day, then don't be stupid and have three shakes. This should go without saying, really.

Creatine monohydrate

This is an absolute classic supplement in the world of sports performance. There is an extraordinary amount of science attesting to its effectiveness – several hundred studies – and it is remarkably cheap. Frankly, you would be crazy not to include it in your plan.

Creatine has been shown to increase power output, increase strength, increase muscle mass (Volek et al., 1999), and increase muscle endurance (although this isn't often its main use) (Chwalbińska-Moneta, 2003), to name just a few. You can see why it would be worth taking, especially when a daily serving will cost as little as five pence! Seriously, for those of you who respond well to creatine (as unfortunately some of you won't), the ROI on that 5p will be amazing.

Several years ago, supplement companies started coming out with new, improved versions, such as creatine ethyl-ester, that promised to work better than the traditional creatine monohydrate, but at a cost. Like most guys, I fell for this and remember thinking it made no difference. Well, a little over ten years later, that has been proven to be the case, so don't fall for the hype. Just buy the basic creatine monohydrate and be done with it. 1kg of the stuff will set you back just £10-12. Bargain.

How to take creatine (you have two options):

1. The traditional way, and the one most products will suggest you do on their labels, is to load it for 5 days at a dose of 20g and then drop to a maintenance dose of 5g per day. That 20g can be divided up equally over 4-5 servings, across the day.

2. Skip the loading phase and go straight to a maintenance dose of 5g per day and ensure you do so for at least a month.

The only real difference, as far as I've seen, is that the loading protocol will saturate the muscle with creatine and therefore increase the amount available to you faster than if you were to skip the loading phase. Loading it will probably bring about the benefits quicker, but those benefits won't be increased by doing so. Therefore, I would choose the option you're more likely to be able to stick to. Adding 20g or 5g of creatine a day to a drink or shake is pretty simple. Let's be honest: both options require you to be consistent, that's all. I'll add that some people experience stomach problems from using creatine in higher doses, again making the non-loading option more appealing to some.

Lastly, creatine will cause weight gain from water retention (within the muscle). This will, of course, be something you'll have to consider if you begin to use this at the start of your diet, and it's just another reason why I recommend you don't use the weighing scales as your only tool for tracking progress.

Coffee (caffeine)

Yes, good old-fashioned coffee. Coffee is a great performance enhancer. If you don't like it, you could just use some caffeine pills. You could also opt for an energy drink – just be sure to get a sugar free one! Coffee used before training or cardio is great, as it will do the following:

- Provide you with energy for the session; it can also improve your performance (Burke, 2008). This is something that many of you will benefit from, especially during busier periods, or if you're having to train first thing in the morning. I hate this, and so I rarely do it, but if "needs must", grab a large espresso, knock it back, and hit the gym hard.

- Caffeine has been shown to acutely enhance strength and power, even in people who are well trained. More strength and power will always lead to better results, and this is a solid reason for using caffeine before training.

- It can speed up your metabolism, meaning you burn more calories per day, and this can aid in your fat loss. The number of calories burned by this metabolism boost is modest at a mere 100 calories, even if consuming 600mg of caffeine (~6 shots of espresso!) (McDonald, 2008), but every little bit helps. Caffeine can also release fatty acids into the bloodstream so that they can then be used as fuel (Kim et al., 2010), making it a great supplement to use before training.

Coffee (or caffeine pills/energy drinks) should be ingested about 30-60 minutes before training, and the recommended dose is ~3-6 mg/kg (Goldstein et al., 2010). So that would be 300-600mg for me. I tend to have 250-300mg, and that seems to be fine for me. As with most things, if you are not used to using caffeine, then start on the lower end and assess how you feel. You can then increase the dose if needed. Personally, I recommend not using these unless you really need to, as habitual coffee drinkers will get used to it and it won't tend to work as well. There is no stimulant that I use before every training session; I simply save them for the times I feel I need them. If I'm dieting, I'll have a coffee prior to cardio, and that's it.

Final thoughts on supplements

This is, of course, not an exhaustive list. As I said at the beginning of this chapter, I primarily wanted to talk about the supplements that I commonly use myself and recommend to clients. I suggest talking to your GP before trying any, and, if you can, getting them to do some blood tests. No point, for example, buying vitamin D3 if your body doesn't need it. If I'm looking to use a new supplement, I will always do my research, and I suggest you do the same. It is not uncommon for supplement companies to make grandiose claims about the "benefits" of a supplement without any research to bolster those claims; or to use something that is backed by research, but then give you a tiny amount of the bloody dose needed to get the benefits.

A great resource, and where I look first, is a website called _www.examine.com._ They can be trusted to give you some impartial advice and the recommended doses. They also show you what research has been done on a particular supplement, and how effective it has been shown to be, in a way that is easy to understand. This makes choosing supplements a lot easier and reduces your chance of getting ripped off. Lastly, before adding any supplements to your plan, do be sure to check that none of them interfere with any medication you might be taking at the time. Get advice on that, just to be on the safe side.

Chapter 3

Effective resistance training made safe and simple

It's time to look at how you should go about doing some safe and effective weight training, even if you're time-poor, a complete novice, or nursing more injuries than the modern-day footballer. Training is often easier to get right – and easier to adhere to – than diet. This is probably due to the fact that training only takes up roughly four to eight hours of your week, whereas controlling what you eat requires effort every hour you are awake.

For many guys, the training part actually becomes pretty enjoyable given some time, and that makes it easier to adhere to, as well. No one ever enjoyed saying no to pizza and beers (but at least it's not forever).

Having worked in gyms for more than a decade, though, I can honestly say that most guys still get this part very, very wrong. If done incorrectly, then at best, you will really slow down results; and at worst, you'll end up injured. Most of you reading this will not be in your 20's, a time where most of us felt indestructible. Sadly, most of you will be at a point where joints creak, muscles ache, and you have a long list of niggles and injuries to keep in mind. It is for this reason that getting the training right is important. One wrong move, one poorly performed rep, and you're laid up in bed nursing a bad back or shoulder injury. Nothing will slow down your progress quite like being "broken", so let's look to avoid that while training with the kind of intensity that will get you the results you are after.

In these coming chapters, I'll aim to go through the main things to consider when creating a training programme, and then offer some examples for you to try.

The benefits - "Why do I need to do some resistance training?"

The goal of a resistance training programme, i.e. weights, is to build muscle and gain strength. Nothing will make you look, feel, and perform better than having more muscle and more strength. I guarantee you that. Bear in mind that inactive adults will have a "3% to 8% loss of muscle mass per decade, accompanied by resting metabolic rate reduction and fat accumulation" (Westcott, 2012). In other words, if you don't hit the gym, age will catch up with you.

Most guys that are new to the gym will mostly be concerned about losing weight. This often means that they have the mentality that their training should be very much focused on calorie burning. This drive to burn calories often leads to participation in fitness classes, or to perform more high-rep circuit based training in the gym. Their goal is to lose fat, but going to the gym to burn fat is shortsighted, and may mean they'll fail to get the benefits of lifting some iron.

My point is that lifting weights in order to gain some strength should be your priority. This is especially true for those of you who have a limited amount of time to train, or for those weeks when you're busier than normal. If in doubt, go and lift some weights. The benefits to resistance training are numerous and will beat doing cardiovascular training, like running and cycling, hands down.

The benefits of resistance training include:

- Increased bone density and strength
- Increased flexibility
- Lower risk of diabetes
- Better mood and wellbeing
- Increase in metabolism
- Reduced blood pressure
- Improved quality of life
- Look better (Duh!)
- Improved mobility
- Less pain and stiffness
- Improved posture
- Improved fat burning and fat loss maintenance
- Better nutrient partitioning (calories go to muscle, not fat)

(Winett and Carpinelli, 2001)

Can we then agree that lifting weights is the way to go, and leave the fitness classes for cardio bunnies? Excellent. Let's break down how to actually create a training programme.

Training frequency

When we are discussing "training frequency", we can actually be talking about two different aspects of training. Both are worth covering. I'm strictly speaking about resistance training here, and not the addition of aerobic exercise.

These two factors are:

1. How many days per week you train
2. How many times you train a specific muscle per week

"How many days per week should I train?"

When thinking about setting up your training plan, the first thing you must ask yourself is: how many days can I realistically train each week? From experience, I'd say that it's fairly common for guys to believe that you must train 5-6 days per week. In my opinion, that is not only overkill for most guys, but for someone running a business and looking after a family, it's simply unrealistic. You can reap the benefits I've stated above by doing just two sessions of 15-20 minutes each week (Winett and Carpinelli, 2001). Consider this the bare minimum needed to get some *health benefits*. However, I'm going to assume you want to transform your physique, as well, and that is going to require a little more work. Not loads, though.

My client Paul has seen fantastic results over the past four years with me, doing just two sessions of 60 minutes per week. Could he improve faster if we added a third session? Sure, I believe so, but he's happy with the balance of gym time to benefits, and so there is no need to change this plan. To a certain extent, there is definitely a dose-response to resistance training, although there is definitely an upper limit for everyone, which we'll cover later on.

Everyone I'm working with at the moment is currently doing three to four resistance training sessions per week, averaging 45-60 minutes. Not a huge time commitment, especially with some of them training at home when it's convenient to them. I feel everyone can find three to four hours for training per week. As my client, Jon once said, "As a business owner, you should be able to make your training and health a priority. I plan my day around my training, NOT the other way around". It's always worth remembering that your health should be your priority.

"How many times should I train each muscle per week?"

The amount of times that you train a muscle is actually pretty important, and it's something that many guys new to the gym will get wrong. It's easy to get it wrong, especially given that many training programmes touted in popular magazines and websites follow the types of programmes that professional bodybuilders use. I made the mistake of following the training programmes of the pros for over 10 years, until I finally decided that there must be a better way. Traditionally (but not always, of course), bodybuilders will train each muscle group just once per week. For example, you may train your chest on a Monday (hence why Monday is often jokingly referred to as "international chest day" in gyms). Most guys just can't wait to hit the bench press.

Training your muscles just once a week is known as "low frequency training". A common training plan for the week would look something like:

- Monday - chest + triceps
- Tuesday - rest day
- Wednesday - back + biceps
- Thursday - rest day
- Friday - legs and calves
- Saturday - shoulders + abs
- Sunday - rest day

With "high frequency training", you'll usually train a muscle two to four times per week. High frequency training programmes will more often be referred to as "full body training", because you need to train multiple muscle groups to fit it all in during a given week. This may look something like:

- Monday - full body
- Tuesday - rest day
- Wednesday - full body
- Thursday - rest day
- Friday - upper body only
- Saturday - lower body only
- Sunday - rest day

Note: The example above is currently what I'm following, and is taken from a great ebook called Fortitude Training by Dr. Scott Stevenson.

As I've said, the most common training frequency seems to be the standard, which is to train each muscle once per week. From experience with myself and my clients, I can say that I believe higher frequency training to be superior for most people. There isn't much research to back it up, but a meta-analysis done by Brad Schoenfeld et al concluded that "...when comparing studies that investigated training muscle groups between one to three days per week on a volume-equated basis, the current body of evidence indicates that frequencies of training twice a week promote superior hypertrophic outcomes to once a week. It can therefore be inferred that the major muscle groups should be trained at least twice a week to maximise muscle growth" (Schoenfeld, Ogborn, and Krieger, 2016). In other words, train large muscle groups at least twice a week if you want them to grow as big as possible.

For most beginners, it's in your best interest to train your muscles more frequently. This allows you to practice and perfect exercises that will most likely be new to you. With my own clients, I'll often start them on a full body training programme that they repeat three to four times a week for that very reason. I'm going to cover this later in this section and offer a basic plan to start you off.

Training volume – "Sets? What are they?

Firstly, when we refer to the amount of "sets" performed for an exercise, what we are talking about is simply how many times you repeat that exercise. For example, if I said I want you to do some push-ups until you fail, then repeat that one more time, that would be two sets. Usually, you will be told to do a certain amount of "working sets". Working sets are simply the main sets you do that are the hardest ones to complete. Therefore, they do not count your warm-up sets. This is important gym lingo to know.

Back to training volume, then. Training volume, with regards to resistance training, is the total number of working sets that you perform on a particular muscle over a period of one week. For example, you might do two exercises for your chest with two working sets each. This would give you four total work sets on your chest for that workout.

This will typically look like this in your plan:

A. Barbell bench press - two sets of 10 reps
B. Pushups - two sets of 10 reps

If you repeated that same session two more times over the week (three times in total), then your total volume for chest that week would be twelve sets.

Training volume is an important variable if your goal is to build muscle, as there is a dose-dependent relationship between the amount of sets performed and how much muscle you'll build. For those of you who are very busy and can't dedicate much time to the gym, the good news is that even low volume (less than five total sets per week per muscle group) will build some muscle, just not loads. (Schoenfeld, 2017). For times when you are busier than usual, like while travelling for business, it's great to know that you can do a little less training than usual and not fear going backwards. In fact, you can still build some muscle! You could probably achieve this in 2 x 1-hour sessions per week, or 3 x 30- to 45-minute sessions.   At the end of the day, maintaining muscle is far easier than building it!

However, it's important to know that more volume will create more muscle. Another meta-analysis by Schoenfeld et al found that performing 10+ sets per muscle group produced almost double the amount of muscle mass that performing 5 or less sets did (Schoenfeld, Ogborn and Krieger, 2016). This means that for those of you who want to *really* improve your physiques to the best of your abilities, you'll need to find that extra bit of time in the gym for those extra sets.

At the time of this writing, only up to 10 or more sets per muscle group has been tested with no upper limit established. However, I've had many clients as high as 20+ sets per week who have done well. Some have not done as well. While some of you reading this will be able to hit muscles with 20 sets per week while making progress, others will find even 10 sets per week a challenge. This will be especially true for those of you who travel a lot, don't get much sleep, and in general feel quite stressed – all of which will affect your ability to recover from the training.

The best thing to do is experiment. This is another reason why I'm big on clients following set programmes and tracking them, rather than going into the gym and randomly just "liftin' shit" ad hoc. If you follow x amount of sets per muscle group for several weeks and track it, you'll be able to gauge how well you're recovering and then adjust accordingly. This is no different to what we've discussed in the diet section. The goal is to be able to tailor make your own plan based on the results you get.

Repetitions: "Should I do high reps for weight loss and definition?"

The word "repetitions" simply describes how many times you perform a particular exercise or lift a weight. If you did 10 pushups, that would be 10 repetitions, which will always be abbreviated to reps. That should be obvious, but you'd be surprised by how many times I've had to explain it over the years.

It is important that you know what the ideal rep range is for you, as many don't really know what is correct. There are typically two main rep ranges that men will use in the gym.

1. They'll stick to the common "three sets of 10 reps" on every exercise. This is not the worst thing you can do, but as you'll learn, sticking to this rep range can cause some problems and may stop you getting optimal results.

2. It's also common to hear of men performing a very high number of reps, like 20+, or simply performing however many reps they can in a set period of time, like in a circuit class (usually one minute). This is their choice because they believe that higher rep training is better for toning up their muscles and losing fat.

The average man who wants to lose weight, improve his health, and look better tends to view their goal not as muscle building, but instead "muscle toning". I'm not sure where the whole "toning" philosophy came from, but it's certainly stuck well! You guys need to stop seeing building muscle and toning as different outcomes. They are not. They are the same thing. So, regardless of whether you told me you wanted to tone your body or build some muscle, your programme would be the same.

How many reps should you do, then? Muscles can grow from placing a load on them and creating tension (heavy sets), as well as by causing metabolic damage (that horrid pump and burn you get from exercise). This means that you can't simply choose one rep scheme, like I stated above in point number one. You will need to work your muscles through reps of six all the way up to 30 (you could go higher, but this can become very time consuming). Personally, I perform reps from six to 25.

You will be best served by performing some of your sets in the lower rep ranges (6-12) and then some in the upper rep ranges (15+). This will tick all of the boxes for optimal muscle growth. The key to successful muscle growth, with any rep range, is reaching "failure" (or getting very close) during a set (Schoenfeld, 2017). Failure is where you can't perform another repetition with quality technique. This is something that's important, especially for higher rep sets that tend to burn so much it hurts. Many will give up before failure, because they've not yet developed the mental strength to endure the pain.

There are some advantages to knowing this. One is that you now have no excuses when you're travelling and need to use a hotel gym. Often, the hotel gym or fitness suite is nothing more than a room with a treadmill and a few light dumbbells. If you're lucky, you might get some machines and cables. This will force you to be creative with your programmes at times. Sure, you might not be able to do squats, deadlifts, and rows; however, you can at least do a workout that utilises lighter weights and higher reps, knowing that they are still worthy of your time. This way, you cannot use the gym's limitations as an excuse to not bother.

Speaking of squats and deadlifts, many of you, like a lot of my clients, will be nursing old injuries that have to be considered. Several of my current clients started with some shoulder pain (although most are pain free now), and so they literally couldn't do lower rep training on them. This was not an issue. Instead, I just programmed exercises they found comfortable, and performed higher reps. As their injuries improved, we gradually began to increase the weights and reduce the reps.

Bottom line is this: work hard across all rep ranges, from six all the way to 30, and you will be fine. It's also a LOT less boring than sticking to the usual "3 sets of 10 reps" – that gets boring really fast.

Tempo: "Some people lift the weights fast, and some slow. Which is right?"

I'm not going to go all "sciencey" on this one, but I did want to cover lifting tempo briefly. If I had a pound for every guy I've seen in the gym aimlessly throwing weights around like he was having an epileptic fit, I'd not need to write this book. Remarkably often, I see guys in the gym who just seem to think swinging weights around will get the job done. It won't, I assure you.

There are many good reasons to control the speed at which you perform your reps. Firstly, it's a lot safer. As I've stated before, most of you reading this will be slightly older. In all likelihood, you'll also have some old injuries just waiting to rear their ugly heads at the first hint of a crappy rep. One bad rep and you are laying on the sofa, nursing a bad back or a pulled shoulder. Simply control your weights and you'll reduce the risk a lot.

Secondly, it will give you more chance to think about

what you are doing. This is referred to as the "mind-muscle connection". To put it simply, the body is lazy and likes to be efficient at completing tasks. Your body prefers to make things easier, not harder. But this isn't the goal with resistance training. You are trying to challenge the muscles you are training, aiming to force them to adapt, i.e. get stronger and bigger. The issue for many of you will be that you are learning to lift weights having spent many years sitting, slouching, and generally ruining your posture. This leads to some muscles being very difficult to isolate and "feel".

A good example will be your back muscles. Improving them is essential for improving posture and reducing back pain. If you move the weights fast, without giving much thought to *how* you should be performing the exercise, you'll end up using other muscles, like the biceps (top of arm) and the upper shoulders and neck (not good if you suffer with neck issues!).

How fast should we lift, then? My advice would be to aim to be as explosive as possible when you lift the weight (known as the concentric phase of the rep). Bear in mind that as the weight gets heavier, the slower it will move, regardless of how fast you try to move it. It's like trying to push a car. No matter how hard you push it, it'll move slowly. As long as it moves, you are fine. As you lower the weight (known as the eccentric phase of the rep), it's worth taking two to three seconds to do this. Make the most of this phase! There are many strength and size benefits to be had from doing so. Too many guys simply let the weight drop under gravity. Resist the temptation to be one of them, and control that weight. This isn't something I'd be too anal about. Just get into the habit of moving weights with control while focusing on the muscle you're trying to target, and you'll be fine.

Rest periods: "How long should I rest between sets?"

The time that you rest in between working sets is important. Rest too long and you'll lose intensity, but don't rest enough and you'll risk not being able to lift the weight you are about to lift in subsequent sets.

Ultimately, what answers this question all boils down to what rep range you are using.

Moderate weight/low rep sets (6-12)

If you are performing heavier weights for lower reps in the 6-12 range, then your goal is to keep the weight as heavy as possible in all sets. At the time of writing this, my heavy back days have rack pulls at a weight of 280kg – almost three times my body weight. My goal is to add some reps or increase the weight I lift every time I repeat this exercise (in rare cases, you might get both). These sets are very demanding! My heart rate will rocket to ~170-180 beats per minute, and I'll be left very breathless. Therefore, it makes sense that in order to achieve my goals on those sets, I would need enough time to recover. I usually take three minutes (and yes, I time that). Two minutes has been shown to be better for muscle growth than a single minute (Schoenfeld et al., 2016), but in my opinion, for those all-out killer sets, three minutes is more favourable. If you need longer, so be it. Just be consistent from week to week.

I will sometimes rest for just two minutes for exercises that are less demanding, but still within this rep range. Exercises done on machines are a good example. With experience, you will soon learn which exercises need that extra recovery.

Light weight/high rep sets (15+)

When using lighter weights for higher reps (15+), you can usually recover faster. Also, the goal of these types of sets is to create a good "pump" in the muscle. Therefore, shorter recovery times work well here.

In these circumstances, I usually rest around 60-90 seconds. I would advise against going below one minute for your recovery, though, as you still don't want to reduce the reps and weight too much – even if the main goal is to pump the muscle up.

The bottom line is that there needs to be a certain amount of recovery to maintain good performance, and to build as much muscle as possible. Remember, when I'm talking about lifting weights, this is my main focus. I would recommend keeping this variable consistent by timing your rest periods. You might think that resting two to three minutes on heavy sets and one to two minutes on light sets would feel like plenty, but there will be times where you're tired, sore, or out of breath. At these times, without the strict limitations of a stopwatch, you could easily rest much longer and not realise it. As with most things, keep yourself accountable. If your time is up and you don't feel ready to lift again, then take a deep breath, man up, and get on with it. This will also help you to be certain that you are improving because you're stronger, and not because you rested longer, which gives a false sense of progress.

Exercise selection: "What is better, free weights or machines?"

The debate about whether free weights like barbells are "better" than machines and cables is one that has been going on for years, and it's ridiculous. As I've alluded to in this whole book, speaking in absolutes when it comes to training and nutrition is stupid. There are far too many factors to consider to be able to make such black and white recommendations. My take on it is that both free weights and machines have their pros and cons, and that some context is certainly needed to decide which is going to be better specifically for you.

Let me break down some of the pros and cons of each for you:

Free weights – pros and cons

Pros

- They allow you to do full movement patterns. For example, you can learn to perform squats correctly. Learning these types of movements translates well into the kind of activities needed in real life.

- Without the additional support of the machine, stabilising muscles and the core are working harder. This will help you develop better posture, balance, and overall strength. This can help to keep the joints healthy, and reduce issues like back pain.

- The movement can be more natural. When using a machine, you are stuck moving the way the machine is designed to move. For some, this can be uncomfortable and aggravate injuries. Differences in height and limb length often make free weight exercises feel better.

- More variety and freedom. Many of my clients train at home, and therefore have neither the space nor the budget to kit out their home gym like a proper gym. Having a set of dumbbells and a barbell with a bench allows you to do a full body workout with minimal kit while needing minimal space. Learning to train with free weights means it's much easier to keep training while you're travelling, as you'll never know what you might get at the hotel gym.

- More efficient. Consider what muscles get worked when performing something like a squat. It's practically a whole-body exercise, certainly when compared with using the leg press at the gym, which isolates just the legs. For the same time, performing both exercises, you can simply get more done. For those of you that are busy, this is an excellent reason to choose free weights over the machines.

Cons
- It takes longer to master free weight exercises. Again, let's use the squat as an example. The squat may take several months for someone to learn and feel comfortable doing, especially with heavier weights. On the other hand, you can get someone on a leg press, and within one to two weeks have them lifting weights that are challenging for them, and importantly, they feel safe doing.

- Far easier to get wrong. The movements are more complex and there is the whole issue of being able to maintain good posture. It's therefore far easier to get wrong, and this risks you wasting time – or worse, injuring yourself.

- You need a spotter. A "spotter" is someone who stays close to you during an exercise, and in the event that you can't complete a rep, will help you finish it and re-rack the weight safely. They also will help you "lift" the weight up. I recently had a client comment that doing the chest press with dumbbells with 12kg had got too easy. Yet, they simply couldn't lift the 14kg on their own to try the new weight. They train alone, and this is a real problem for free weights. Many of you will also train alone and come across this issue.

- They challenge your core, abs, and posture more. Yes, I know this was also listed as a pro, but it can easily become a con as well. Let's imagine on Monday you have challenged yourself to do some heavy squats. You go to train Wednesday, and find that your abs and core are still fatigued. This would make doing more free weight exercises difficult. Doing so would also further fatigue those same muscles. This fatigue would make you weaker, and this is certainly not advantageous.

Machines and cables – pros and cons

Pros

- They are simple to use. Once things (such as the seat height) have been adjusted and are correct for your body, then you are ready to go. Simply place the "pin" on the weight you desire and lift. Most machines aren't used for complex movements, and this makes them easier to learn and gain confidence on.

- You can learn to isolate and feel muscles easily. I touched upon this in the tempo section, that some muscles will feel very hard to train – like your brain isn't connected to them. Machines provide a simple way to learn how to do this without having to concentrate on lots of complex movements. ALL new clients start much of their sessions on the machine in the first several weeks, so I can assess how they move and get their feedback.

- You rarely need a spotter. Machines are very safe to challenge yourself on, without the fear of dropping a dumbbell on your face. I usually find new clients are more inclined to get the intensity high enough to get results in the early days.

- They are safer. For a start, on most machines you won't lift as heavy, and this reduces the risk of doing any damage. They are great for training areas of the body where you lack confidence or may have had previous injuries.

Cons
- The movement can be restrictive. Bear in mind, you can only move the way in which the machine is designed to do so. Some machines will simply have a movement path that won't agree with the way in which your body moves. This can make exercises uncomfortable. A good example is shoulder pressing above the head. Many of my clients come to me with a rounded, slouched posture from years of sitting behind a desk. They tend to need to push the weights slightly forward of the body, as they simply don't have the flexibility to get the arm behind them any further. However, many shoulder press machines will require that amount of flexibility to be used. In this circumstance, that particular machine is best avoided, and an alternative exercise found.

- No real use of your postural muscles. Machines will usually have a nice, comfy pad to sit on, and often even a back rest to lean against. They require very little use of your stabilising muscles and core, simply because you are so supported. This is not advantageous if you specifically want to improve your postural strength and reduce back pain.

- You don't train full movements. Instead of learning to perform exercises like squats and deadlifts, which cross over well into everyday life, you end up just training isolated muscles. Although it never hurts to have stronger muscles, it's useful to be able to learn to use those muscles together while moving, rather than in isolation.

- You need to join a gym. Some of you may not want to join a gym or feel that you don't have the time. Machines are expensive, and therefore the likelihood of having all the machines needed for a full training session in a home gym is very small – unless you are willing to invest a lot of money, and you have space for them.

- The machines get very busy in commercial gyms, especially at peak times. If you only know how to use one particular machine, for example, for your chest, and the gym you use only has one of those machines, then you run the risk of your session taking way more time than it should do. For most of you, you simply won't want to hang around waiting for someone to finish up.

Practical recommendations

With all that in mind, what do I recommend? Well, really, it depends on you. If you're a beginner, or even returning to training after a long period off, then you are going to want to focus mostly on getting the exercises correct, getting used to "feeling" certain muscles, and ensuring your training has some intensity. It therefore makes sense to do a large proportion of your training with machines and cables. There are simply too many advantages to doing so.

However, that doesn't mean you must do all your exercises on them. At some point, you're going to have to perform some free weight exercises, or you'll never master them. Something that I might do with my clients is give them a free weight exercise to use as a warm-up. This gives them a chance to get the body warmer, while practicing the technique. Of course, this would be done with a light weight. After that is complete, they would essentially "finish off" that particular muscle with a machine, knowing it's safe to work hard. Over a period of several weeks, that warm-up exercise would eventually become their first exercise due to the progress they have naturally made with it. This will ultimately depend on how long it takes you to learn the exercise, and gain confidence with it.

For example, training legs might look something like this:

A. Goblet squat - 4-6 sets of 15-20 reps with a light weight, focusing on control and technique. No need to fail the sets. If possible, film this for evaluation.

B. Leg press - 2 sets of 12-15 - fail last set
C. Leg curl - 2 sets of 10-12 - fail last set

As you can see, exercise A is simply to practice and learn a squat movement. It gets the whole body nice and warm, as well, which is a nice bonus. Once this is over, though, the more intense part of the session starts.

Several weeks later, this might look more like:

A. Goblet or front squat - 2 sets of 6-10 reps - fail both sets
B. Leg press - 2 sets of 12-15 - fail both sets
C. Leg curl - 2 sets of 10-12 - fail both sets

Notice how exercise A is no longer simply a practice exercise. Over the preceding weeks, the person has developed a better understanding of the exercise, and is confident enough to do it with heavier weights. It has become a main exercise. This is simply how exercises evolve over time. There is no rush with the learning process. It is better to take your time and be safe than risk getting injured.

For those of you who are beginners, I **<u>strongly</u>** recommend you invest in a good coach. Don't be that guy who clearly has no clue what he's doing in the gym. A good coach will reduce the learning curve by months. Think of the cost of not investing in someone to coach you. There's the wasted time, the frustration, and the fact that a large percentage of you won't achieve the level of results you expect without a coach. As my client Jon explained in the foreword.

It's also possible that in the long run, not having a coach will cost you more. No, seriously. You can waste money on a gym membership you don't use. The cost of fixing injuries sustained while not training effectively isn't cheap. Then there's the cost to your business of not having the motivation and the energy to be as productive as you could be. Investing several thousand in your health will get you a huge ROI, I guarantee it. I see it time and time again with my own clients.

It's more difficult to make recommendations for those of you who are already training, and just feel you should be getting more from it. It's very common for me to get a client who fits this description, and for me to then see that they are doing everything wrong. Basically, they are a beginner who just so happens to have been going to the gym longer. This happens a LOT. If this is you (you'll need to be very honest with yourself here), then go back and follow the steps laid out for the beginner. Start from scratch, get some help, and then move forward.

I think it's very common for men to overcomplicate everything. The gym is no different. Let's use myself as an example. Even with all my experience and knowledge, my training is very simple. I'll use the leg day again as an example so you can compare it to the example laid out above for the beginner:

A. Barbell squat - 2 sets of 6-8 - fail last set only
B. Barbell stiff leg deadlift - 1 sets of 8-10 - fail set
C. Leg extension machine - 1 sets of 12 reps - fail set
D. Calf raises - 3 sets of 6-12 reps - fail all sets
E. Adductor machine (the inner thigh machine that the ladies love) - 1 set of 15-20 reps - fail set

There isn't a lot of difference. I have two free weight exercises than will fatigue my lower back and core. Therefore, I then switch to machines to further challenge my legs without tiring my back out more. Most people overcomplicate things. It really doesn't need to be rocket science.

Here are some general rules to help you:

1. If you have injuries, try using a machine and go light. This way, you can learn to "work around" the area giving you trouble.

2. If you struggle to "feel" a muscle work – by which I mean that it doesn't feel like the exercise is doing anything – then find a machine that isolates that muscle and practice.

3. If you are new to a free weight exercise, go slow and use light weights. Do more sets so that you can master the

movement, and consider using it as a way of warming up.

4. If you have poor posture that has led to neck and back pain, then use the machines to begin strengthening the muscles that have become weak. This is where a good coach is worth his weight in gold.

5. If you get to the gym and your core, abs, and/or lower back are fatigued from a previous session, then consider using more machines to allow those areas to recover. Once recovered, go back and try the free weight exercises again.

6. If short on time, consider using both. I like to sometimes do a machine exercise. Then, instead of resting between sets, I'll use some free weights or body weight to do another exercise (usually a different muscle group). A good example would be to do leg presses and push-ups together. This is known as a "superset".

Deloads and time off – "When should I take some time off to rest?"

It's all very well training your arse off week in, week out, but a point will come when that hard training will begin to take its toll on your body. For this reason, it's important to take a step back occasionally to allow your body to recover. This a known as either a "deload phase" or simply as good old-fashioned time off, depending on how you do it.

I'm including a section on this because many will get to the point where they need to deload, and then simply ignore it. Some will do so because they are enjoying the training and don't want to stop; some are scared of going backwards; and others may do so because they simply don't know it's okay to rest! I've known many men who have had a "Sod it, I'll push through it" attitude, and sadly made things worse for themselves.

This is something I've experienced time and time again with my own clients. One of the questions on the check-in form they must answer weekly is: "When was your last deload?". I would say that 80% of the time, someone's first check in will say something like "Haven't done one", or, my favourite, "What is a deload?". It's therefore evident that most guys need to be educated about deload phases so that they can take advantage of them.

Once you are at the point where you are training intensely, especially while dieting, a deload works very well for many reasons. For most men, if you are not missing sessions and you are heading into the gym focused on beating the lifts you did the previous week, it won't usually take more than six to eight weeks before you start to see and feel the signs that you need to recover.

Signs that you need a deload:
- Joints can start to hurt
- You begin to pick up injuries or old ones return
- Motivation decreases
- Strength improvements slow down, stop or even regress
- Sleep is worse than usual
- You begin to pick up bugs and colds a little easier
- You feel sorer after training than usual, and recovery takes longer
- You have a poorer than usual appetite

Through experience, you will soon learn to listen to your body and know when to take a deload.

How to deload

You really have two choices when it comes to deloads. You can take some time off fully from the gym, anywhere up to a full week; or you can carry on training, but make some adjustments to your programme to ensure that you can recover.

My thoughts on this are that if you've really beat yourself into the ground by training hard, doing cardio, along with work and other life stresses, and you've powered through a few more weeks than you should have, then take a full five to seven days off. Remember, I said there were some common "symptoms" to look out for; well, if you've ignored them, then you will want some full time off.

I don't feel this is the optimal choice. As Dr. Scott Stevenson[13] points out in his training ebook, Fortitude Training, if you maintain how hard you train (intensity)

during a deload, then you can maintain all the strength you gained before backing off (Ratamess et al., 2003) – even if you train fewer times per week than usual. Remember that the goal is to be able to take some time off from the gym to recover <u>without</u> losing any of the progress you'd made.

Therefore, upon returning to training, you should reach new limits. Think of this approach as *two steps forward; half a step back; repeat.*

Let's discuss the second approach, where you carry on training. To do this correctly, you have to maintain your

---

13   Dr. Scott Stevenson, PhD, is an applied exercise physiologist and competitive bodybuilder with over 20 years of experience as a personal trainer. I used his programme for my own training and can't speak highly enough of him.

intensity (how hard you work) while allowing some recovery time. This is achieved by doing the following:

1. Reducing the volume per muscle group. We've already discussed training volume in a previous section, so you should understand that I simply mean doing fewer sets on each muscle than normal. I usually reduce my training volume by 50%. This means that if you usually do a total of 12 sets on your chest each week, you would reduce that to just 6 sets.

2. Reducing the number of days you train that week (simply going to the gym less) is, of course, going to give you more recovery days. I usually reduce this by just one day. Most of you will be going three to four days per week in the gym, and so this would simply mean doing two to three instead.

3. Reduce the amount of weight you lift. During the deload, don't do any of your normal heavy lifts in the 6-12 rep range. Instead, reduce the weights and go for reps of 20-30.

4. Maintain your intensity. This means still hitting those sets hard, and failing them as usual. This is fine. The reduced amount of work you do over the whole week will be enough to allow for recovery.

The cool thing here is that research also shows that you can maintain your progress even when you can't train as frequently or with weights as heavy as usual; for example, when travelling for business. In fact, you could use this strategy during the times when you are busier than usual, knowing that it won't set you back.

Example -

	Normal training	Deload training
Days per week	3	2
Number of sets	15	8
Reps performed	6-30	20-30
Intensity	Fail sets	Fail sets

This section won't necessarily become relevant at first, while you are in a phase at the gym based mostly on learning and building confidence. You might not need to deload for 8-12 weeks for this reason. However, keep it in mind for the when the time does time so you are prepared.

Key points -

1. Look for signs of fatigue, soreness, lack of motivation, disturbed sleep, and regressing strength after 6-8 weeks.
2. When you start to notice these symptoms, then it's time to take a step back.
3. Reduce the amount of days you're training by one.
4. Reduce the total amount of hard sets you are doing by 50%.
5. Maintain the intensity by still lifting your normal weights, but only in the 20-30 rep range.

Muscle soreness – "I wasn't very sore. Maybe I didn't work hard enough?"

Muscle soreness. I'm sure every one of you reading this has experienced it at some point in your life. It's a perfectly normal response to exercise, and isn't something to be concerned about. "Delayed onset muscle soreness", or DOMS for short, usually starts ~24 hours after training, and looks to be caused by tiny microtears in the muscle fibres (Schoenfeld, 2012). In extreme cases, it can last for several days and be very painful. In my first year as a personal trainer, I had a client that I trained a little too hard on her first session. That session resulted in her having to take *two days* off work! Yep, she was in so much pain she couldn't leave the bed. Don't worry, I never made that mistake again, but it does go to show you what can go wrong if you overdo your training, especially in the beginning.

One issue related to muscle soreness is that it's extremely common for men to train with the goal of getting sore in mind. They like to use how sore they are to judge whether they had a good training session. I'll admit, it's nice to have a little soreness after a good session, but it shouldn't be overly painful.

There are a couple of reasons why training specifically to create soreness isn't productive. Firstly, as I've already explained, you should be aiming to train muscles multiple times per week. This will be difficult if, after every session, you are sore for several days. Therefore, being able to recover fast enough to train again is essential. Secondly, being sore doesn't equate to improvement. Simply experiencing soreness doesn't mean that you're creating stronger, larger muscles. In fact, I rarely get very sore, but I've still managed to grow fairly well over the years.

I see the same with many of my clients. Rarely do I ever push them so hard that they are crippled for a week. Again, they improve just fine. I've also had plenty of clients over the years come to me bragging about how much soreness their "amazing" training programme causes them, and yet they don't look that great. I've also noted over the years that some muscle groups just don't get as sore as others. For me personally, I rarely get very sore shoulders, no matter how much I train them. My triceps (back of the upper arm) are also pretty resilient to muscle soreness; yet again, they've grown.

There is also a genetic aspect to it, as well, where some people just get sorer than others. This is most likely also related to the fact that some people recover from exercise better than others. This will also need to be considered. We do need to create muscle damage in order for that muscle to rebuild itself bigger and stronger, so a bit of soreness could be considered a good thing. Still, I feel that this isn't a great reason to aim to be excessively sore. Some soreness is fine, and most people like to feel like they've "done something" after the gym. Even I do, but not to the extent where I have to cautiously sit on the toilet like I'm 90 years old. I draw the line at being that sore. Science backs all this up as well. A great article called "Is Postexercise Muscle Soreness a Valid Indicator of Muscular Adaptations?" concluded that "The applicability of DOMS in assessing workout quality is inherently limited, and it therefore should not be used as a definitive gauge of results" (Schoenfeld and Contreras, 2013).

I feel I should state the obvious, just in case, and remind you that IF you're returning to exercise after many years of being inactive (or having never exercised), you will be sore in the beginning. The newbie trainer will often experience soreness far greater than what their training programme would predict to cause, but this soon improves.

In conclusion, you don't need to be whining about how sore you are to anyone who will listen in order to improve. As I've said before, some soreness is fine, and to many people, it feels great; but don't be led to believe that it's a must. Ultimately, your best way to gauge improvements is to stand naked in front of the mirror and ask yourself if you're looking better, while looking at the weights you are lifting and ensuring they are increasing.

The Logbook – "Is it important for me to record my training sessions?"

A logbook is simply where you are going to record everything you do in the gym, so that you can reference it the next time that you go. Returning to using a logbook to record my training sessions is one of the simplest yet most productive things I've done for my training in the past few years. At some point over the past few years, I got complacent and stopped using this valuable tool. In the early days, when I began training at around the age of 16, I religiously recorded literally every rep of every session. In fact, I've still got many of those books.

The obvious reason for writing down what you have lifted during a gym session is simply so you know what you are trying to beat the next time you train. Most guys will remember their best lifts for a handful of exercises, often the ones they like and are progressing well with. For example, most guys will remember their best bench press. That doesn't mean you will remember everything you do, especially if you're doing different exercises every session and therefore won't repeat an exercise for several days.

The other, not-so-obvious reason to record your lifts is

for accountability. There will come a point where you'll head into the gym, and you'll look at your logbook, and the session you are about to do will make you anxious. This is because you know that what's in store is going to be difficult. Lifting weights you've never experienced before really can be quite intimidating. My client Jon is experiencing this himself. At the age of 51, he's lifting weights that he wasn't able to do in his 30's! Jon's sessions scare the shit out of him, BUT the progress he is making is phenomenal. The same can be said of <u>all</u> my clients who embrace the logbook, and the challenge of trying to beat it, week in, week out.

You won't change your body if you're always hiding in your comfort zone – and hiding in your comfort zone is very easy to do. Truth be told, I did this for the first seven or eight years of my training. I'm no psychologist, but for me, I find that if I can see what weights and reps I am supposed to do in a session in black and white, I'm more likely to actually do it. I feel like I can't back out. For some reason, if I don't have the book to "tell me" what I *should be lifting*, my mind starts to play tricks on me and I look for reasons NOT to attempt those personal bests. Thoughts like "I'm too sore today" or "I'm too tired today" start to creep into my head – but they're nothing more than excuses to try and not put myself into a situation that I know won't be pleasant. My logbook makes me do it. It may seem strange, and yet I've heard many other people say similar things. I strongly recommend you listen to this piece of advice because getting stronger over time is what's going to change your body shape in the quickest possible time. Here is a photo of an old logbook I found:

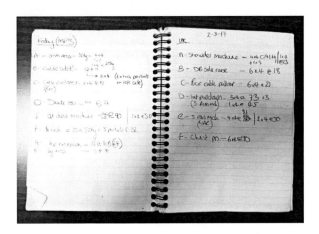

Yeah, it's a little scruffy, but creating a masterpiece is the last thing on my mind during training. What I'm recording is the following information:

- The order in which I performed my exercises, as changing this affects the weights you can lift. Something performed first will always be better than if it's performed last.

- The weight I used for my main sets

- The reps I managed to perform for those main sets

- Sometimes I add a note. For example, if I'm feeling overly tired, or I can feel an injury creeping in, I'll comment about this so that the next time I look at those records I know why something might look "off".

This is very simple. Get a book and pen, or use your phone and download a fitness app. The next time you attempt an exercise, find out what you are trying to beat, and go for it.

Key points -

- Buy a small logbook. I recommend getting a durable one so it doesn't fall apart and you lose pages.

- Record the exercise you do for every session and the reps and sets for that particular exercise.

- Even if you think you'll remember it all, you won't. Believe me.

- Having your session written out and knowing what you need to achieve in the session prior to starting will add some accountability.

Putting it all together to create a plan

In the previous sections, I have broken up and explained to you all the main variables of resistance training. Over time, you will learn and apply these to your own training more and more. There is a risk that at this point, your head will be spinning with information overload. This would not surprise me. However, please remember that you're not meant to be able to learn all of this in one fell swoop. In the real world, you'll learn a piece of it, apply it in training, make some mistakes, and then return to the book. You will need to return to this book many times, each time learning something new about training that didn't sink in before, and then get back into the trenches ready to give it a go.

Having said that, I think that it's a good idea that I put all the pieces together for you and provide you with a plan that the majority of you will be able to try right away. Let's take all the information from all of the resistance training sections prior to this one, and then apply it. I would recommend you choose to do a full body training programme that's performed three to four times per week. This will allow you to train your muscles several times a week, as well as allowing you to perform similar exercises so that you can learn how to do them well. You could vary each workout by changing an exercise for a variation – for example, pushups change to the bench press or a barbell row to a DB row. If you have no idea what any of those are, then it's okay. I have this covered.

Here is how a three-day training plan would look for those of you who are busier.

Day	Area of the body
Monday	Full body gym training
Tuesday	Rest day or just cardio
Wednesday	Full body gym training
Thursday	Rest day or just cardio
Friday	Full body gym training
Saturday	Rest day or just cardio
Sunday	Rest day

The sessions used in this training week would look like this:

Day 1: Full body session (upper body training first)

	Exercise	SETS (not including warm up sets)	REPS PERFORMED	REST PERIOD
A	GOBLET SQUAT	2	10-12	2-3 mins
B	ROMANIAN DEADLIFT	2	12-15	2-3 mins
C	BENT OVER BARBELL ROW	2	10-12	2-3 mins
D	ASSISTED PULL UP	2	12-15	2-3 mins
E	BENCH PRESS	2	10-12	2-3 mins
F	PEC FLY MACHINE	2	12-15	2-3 mins
G	DB SHOULDER PRESS	2	10-12	2-3 mins
H	CABLE FACE PULL	2	15-20	2-3 mins
I	BARBELL CURL	2	12-15	2-3 mins
J	TRICEP DIPS	2	10-12	2-3 mins

Day 2: Full body session 2 (leg training first)

	Exercise	SETS (not including warm up sets)	REPS PERFORMED	REST PERIOD
A	LEG PRESS	2	10-12	2-3 mins
B	HAMSTRING CURL	2	12-15	2-3 mins
C	SEATED ROW MACHINE	2	10-12	2-3 mins
D	LAT PULL DOWN	2	12-15	2-3 mins
E	DB INCLINE PRESS	2	10-12	2-3 mins
F	DB CHEST FLY	2	12-15	2 mins
G	STANDING OVERHEAD PRESS	2	10-12	2 mins
H	REVERSE PEC DEC	2	15-20	2 mins
I	BICEP CABLE CURL	2	12-15	2 mins
J	CLOSE GRIP BENCH PRESS	2	10-12	2 mins

What I've done here is pretty simple. I've just followed the parameters I've already discussed to create this plan.

- *Training days:* 3 days per week
- *Sets per muscle group:* 12, lowish and should be okay to begin with while weights are going to be fairly light.
- *Rest between sets:* 2-3 minutes depending on how demanding the exercise is.
- *Exercise section:* Combination of free weights and machines, just as an example. This can easily be changed based on your confidence, knowledge and issues such as injuries.
- *Recovery:* A day off in between will be fine for most. This can, of course, be based on how you feel.

This programme focuses on the whole body, and uses exercises that allow you to get stronger, and can be used to create intensity and burn calories. You'll notice that I alternate starting the session between the upper body and the lower body. This is simply so that each one gets a chance to begin the session when you're feeling your most energetic. If, for example, you do legs at the end of the session every time, you will find that area might not progress as fast. This is because, by working on your legs last each time you exercise, you will always be doing those exercises in a fatigued state.

I would simply rotate between those two training programmes over the course of three to four days a week, depending on what your schedule allows you to commit to. You don't have to have just two different training programmes, by the way. There is no reason why you couldn't have three to four different programmes that follow the same basic structure, and do them over the course of a week. Every time you return to do a session again, you would look at your logbook and decide on what weights and reps you need to perform on each exercise to progress from the last time you did it. If you do that over the course of several months, you will get very good at performing those exercises, while at the same time getting fairly strong at them as well. It's a matter of ticking all the boxes to ensure your physique continues to improve over time.

The Bonus

I know what you are thinking... you have no idea what any of those exercises even are, or what they look like! Not to worry. Just visit *www.philagostino.co.uk/bonus* and you can have access to a <u>free</u> resource section that has videos of them all.

Chapter 4

Preparing your body for training

The warm up – "How do I prepare my body for my training session?"

Before you get to the nitty-gritty of a training session, and are attempting to push yourself to the max, you'll need to prepare your body first. This, as you probably already know, is called "the warm up". You are quite literally warming up the body. Warm muscles are more pliable than cold muscles, and therefore the warm up will reduce the risk of injury. Getting warmer also improves the way in which your body will move by increasing the range of motion your joints can move through. Think of how stiff you can feel in the morning. This usually gets worse as we age. For some, it can hurt to move at all. Can you imagine lifting weights when you feel like this? Definitely not! There are other reasons to warm up that I'll discuss as I go through the different ways to warm up.

The aerobic warm-up

As I said above, your body isn't going to perform at its best when it's cold and stiff. If you head to the gym and start loading up bars for lifting, at best, you will feel weak, and at worst, you'll hurt yourself. Therefore, it's a good idea for you to do 5-10 minutes of low intensity exercise on something like the bike or treadmill to raise your body temperature. Typically, you just want to do as long as you need to break into a light sweat and to feel like you're loosening up. Be careful here. You definitely don't want to overdo the duration and the intensity, because it will tire you out and affect the weight training part of your session. Keep it easy and brief.

Stretching

Not the most glamorous part of a training session, especially compared to the fun that can be had lifting weights in the gym, and this is probably why it's often an ignored aspect of the warm up. I've definitely been guilty of skipping this part since I've been bodybuilding, if I'm honest. Although, I don't skip the warm up entirely, as I shall explain in this section. However, back when I was kickboxing I stretched a lot to be able to improve the height of my kicks. This is essential when you're only 5'6" tall. Back then, we did a lot of stretching, and at one point, I could practically get into the box splits (the one where your legs go outwards – think Jean Claude Van Damme doing it with his legs on chairs. Except I never needed the chairs!). The reason for stretching is to improve your muscles' ability to lengthen, which is important in any training programme, because a muscle that doesn't lengthen well will reduce performance and increase the risk of injury.

I'll discuss the two most common types of stretching I advise:

1. **Static stretching** – This is probably the first type of stretching that will come to mind for most of you. It's the type of stretching that involves holding the stretch for a set period of time, usually 15-60 seconds. A good example will be touching your toes to stretch the back of your legs

2. **Dynamic stretching** – Dynamic stretches involve movements that take your body through full ranges of motion in order to stretch the muscles of the joint. There isn't a hold with this type of stretching. A good example, if you wanted to dynamically stretch the hips and legs, would be to do some bodyweight squats. These are done in a controlled manner to slowly lengthen the muscles, preparing them for training.

It's clear that there are some benefits to stretching, but the question that is often asked (and debated) is whether or not it should be performed before or after resistance training – or both – and, also importantly, which type. This is still a fairly controversial subject (Page, 2012). The reason for this debate is that several studies have shown that static stretching before training can reduce performance by reducing power and strength (Taylor et al., 2009). Hardly a good thing! Now, having said that, these studies tend to have people perform fairly lengthy static stretches that don't relate to what you or I would ever do in the real world. They will often also have the participants go straight into a test of strength immediately after the stretching. This, as you will learn, is not how we ever do things in the gym (McDonald, 2008).

Whether you need to stretch prior to lifting weights is probably more dependent on your current needs and limitations. Those you who are fairly injury free, more flexible and, dare I say it, younger will most likely only need a brief stretching protocol prior to the weights section. For this, the American College of Sports Medicine recommends doing static stretches, holding for 10-30 seconds and repeated 3-4 times (Nadelen, 2016) or doing some dynamic stretching. Personally, I have always preferred to do dynamic stretches prior to my warm up sets for my first exercise, which will be discussed in its own section. Those of you who are older, more injured, and struggle with flexibility may want to hold stretches slightly longer, up to 60 seconds. Will it reduce performance? Quite possibly, but a slight reduction in performance is much better than an injury that stops you performing altogether. You can't improve your fitness laid up on the couch with a slipped disc. So, first and foremost, we should aim to reduce the risks as much as possible and prioritise safety. For those of you who need more flexibility, I would recommend stretching after the training session when you're nice and warm.

You guys would also benefit from adding some stretching at other times of the day so you can increase how often you do them. Aim to do this when you're warm; for example, after walking the dog or having had a hot bath to ensure the muscles are ready to be lengthened.

The Bonus

For videos on how to perform some basic stretches, visit www.philagostino.co.uk/bonus and get access to a free resource section.

The specific warm up for resistance training

So far, we've discussed elevating your body temperature and then stretching your muscles. These are both general ways of preparing yourself for resistance training. However, you'll need to do something that's more specific to the task of lifting weights before you can safely and effectively start to push yourself hard. By the time you get to point of actually lifting some weight, you will be feeling warm and more flexible; but there is no way you can just jump to your maximal weight on the bar. Therefore, you'll perform 3-5 warm-up sets, where you gradually increase the weight and reduce the reps, every set getting closer to the weight you have planned for your work sets. This will do a few things. It will allow you to "practice" the technique of that particular lift. This is highly important, and even more so for you guys that are new to compound exercises that demand a lot of control like squats and deadlifts. The warm up sets allow you to remind yourself of how it should look and feel, but while the weight is still low. The warm up sets are also dynamic in nature, and therefore, they will help to further stretch any muscles that might still feel "tight" by increasing blood flow and muscle temperature.

For example, I tend to have fairly tight hips; so on the days that I squat, the first two or three sets, when the weight is low, can feel pretty horrible, and I don't have very good range of motion (I don't get very low!). Gradually, over the course of four or five sets, I loosen up and my depth improves. If I add too much weight before doing this, my technique would be simply fucking awful. Plus, the chance of me getting injured would be much greater.

I also find that warm up sets will help myself, and clients, with any confidence issues we might have when aiming to lift a weight we've never tried before. Let's assume you've never squatted 150kg. Performing sets at 100kg, 120kg and then 140kg should allow you to get a feel for the weight, and therefore be mentally ready to attempt that 150kg. Simply being warmed up, and having done several sets to get focused, will make your training safer and more pleasant.

How to do warm up sets for resistance training

There are a few factors that will determine how you will do this:

1. How complex the exercise is
2. How heavy the work set is that you are working towards
3. Where during the session the exercise is

Briefly then, exercises that are more complex, like a squat or a deadlift, will require more practice sets; and so here I recommend you do as many as you need to do to feel ready to get to the heavier weights. Complex exercises like these will usually (but not always) be done fairly early on in your session, and so using them to get multiple muscles warm and prepared is a great idea. These exercises should also be the ones you lift the most weight on. You might be able to deadlift 150kg while only being able to row 50kg. It's obvious that it will take longer to prepare yourself for the deadlift compared to the row. I tend to begin with ~40-50% of the weight I'm ultimately aiming to achieve and work up the weight gradually. I will also start with fairly high reps and as the weight gets heavier, and I'm closer to my goal, I'll reduce them. This is to save energy for the main set while still allowing me to get a feel for the weight. Let's take a squat with a goal of 180kg, the warm-up would look like so:

Set 1: 10 reps with just the bar,
        briefly holding each rep to stretch
Set 2: 10 reps @ 60kg
Set 3: 10 reps @ 100kg
Set 4: 6-8 reps @ 140kg
Set 5: 4-6 reps @ 160kg
Set 6: 6-12 reps @ 180kg

For some of you, this won't be as relevant (initially) because you'll be newer to many of these exercises, and therefore lifting much lighter weights. If this is the case, then you can still start around 50% and work up the weights; but the main reason for doing this will be purely to practice the movement patterns.

Exercises that are simpler and require much less skill, such as bicep curls, will usually not need as many warm up sets. Consider that these exercises will usually come nearer to the end of a training session; so not only is the movement simpler to perform, but the muscles will already be very warm. For example, if you've done several sets of rows and pull ups for your back, then your arms will be warm already. In this case, I tend to do one or two warm-up sets, and will sometimes not do any. I make that choice based on how I'm feeling.

If I'm about to use a muscle that I struggle to "feel" (most people will have some muscles that just don't naturally tense easily for numerous reasons) then I will definitely do a warm up or two purely to get myself focused on that particular muscle. Here I'll do one or two sets of 10-15 reps, slowly moving the weight as I really concentrate on form. I use the analogy of driving a car a lot for this. Think of how when you first learnt to "pull away", you first had to slowly find the "biting point" of the clutch, and then slowly add the accelerator. This is how I warm up muscles I'm poor at using: moving slowly, finding the tension where it SHOULD be felt, and then I'll add more strength to move the weight.

Many of you will have to use this technique for muscles that get "lazy" from everyday poor posture, such as your bum, back, and abdominals. I'm going to discuss this in more detail in another section, as it's an important aspect of making training effective. These types of exercise will again be relatively light as well. A warm up for something like a tricep extension on the cables, where the goal weight might only be 15kg would simply be:

Set 1: 15 reps @ 7-8kg - done slow, controlled with
    the focus on "feel"
Set 2: 10 reps @ 10-12kg
Set 3: 10-15 reps @ 15kg

Bear in mind this might all change from week to week. One week, you might feel like you're 18 years old again, warm-up easily, and do a great set. The following week is the complete opposite; you're tired, stiff, and feeling a little worn out, and therefore you need far more warm-ups. Learn to listen to your body and take your time.

I'll end by saying DO NOT rush these. I've injured myself a few times over the past 15 years, and I can say that it usually isn't when the weight is at its heaviest, as you might imagine. Why? Because once the weight is heavy, I'm warmer and, more importantly, I'm concentrating on the technique. I remember really screwing my back doing some deadlifts once. I was working up to 180kg, very heavy for me at the time, and in my excitement to get to the fun part, I rushed the warm-ups. I put my back out using just 80kg. Light weights with poor form can still hurt you; and when the weight is light, you're more likely to take it for granted and be slack on form. Be patient and do your warm ups as if every set will be super heavy. This will also get you used to practicing perfect form, and prevent you from getting into bad habits that will increase your risk of doing something wrong once the weight is heavier.

In conclusion, this is something I urge you to trial and error for yourself and find what makes your lifting sessions feel safe and effective as possible.

Example warm up routine for a full body weight training day:

Warm up phase	Exercise	Sets	Time	Notes
Aerobic warm up	Any cardio machine. E.g. bike, treadmill, rowing machine	n/a	5-10 minutes	Not too hard. Just enough to breath heavier and break a sweat
Static stretching	Stretch major muscle groups e.g. backs and fronts of thighs, chest, hips, back, bum and shoulders	2-4	15-30 seconds	Get muscles
Specific warm up	For the first exercise of major muscle groups unless muscles are feeling warm and flexible. E.g. squat for legs, barbell row for back.	3-5 sets gradually increasing the weight	n/a	Start at around 50% of goal weight and slowly work up until ready for heaviest set

Key points -

- The goal of any warm-up routine is to prepare the body for exercise and reduce the risk of injury by raising its core and muscle temperatures.
- The first part of the warm-up is very general, and can be performed on any cardiovascular machine, such as a treadmill, a bike, or a rowing machine until you break a light sweat.
- Once the body and muscles are warm, you can lightly stretch the major muscles of the body to improve your flexibility. This is a good option for those who are older, more prone to injuries, or who suffer with poor flexibility.
- You can perform static stretches that are held for a period of time, or dynamic stretches that involve movements that lengthen and shorten your muscles e.g. lunges or body weight squats.
- A specific warm up can then be performed by using the first exercise of a given muscle group (although some will use several) to further increase range of movement, increase blood flow, and prepare you mentally.
- The exercise used can start at around 50% of your goal weight for about 10 reps. You'll then gradually increase the weight of every set (and reduce the reps) until you feel prepared to hit your goal weight for that session.

Activation exercises

Activation exercises are exercises used with the goal of improving how well you can tense a specific muscle. Some muscles can become difficult to tense, even if you concentrate on them well; especially if they have become overly weak or overly lengthened from poor posture. Great examples include your butt (the gluteus maximus or glutes for short), the muscles that make up your back, and your core. In my first year as a trainer, I qualified as a Pilates instructor – not a bad gig for a 21-year-old man in a time when male instructors were extremely rare, and Pilates classes were attended mostly by bored housewives (but I'll save those stories for another book). For those who aren't familiar with Pilates, it's a system of exercises designed to increase your body's stability, flexibility and control. In other words, it's used to correct the mess we get ourselves into by sitting, driving and slouching for too long.

The thing that almost everyone realises very early on in their first class is that some muscles almost feel nonexistent. Participants would often comment that they would "get" what I was trying to explain to them, but they literally couldn't then execute it. "Tense your bum", I'd say, and then nothing. Not even a twitch. Consider this: if you can't flex a muscle while lying on the floor, what chance will you have when you try to do so with weights? Another example of when I personally realised I struggled with flexing certain muscles was when I first started having posing lessons with a coach for my bodybuilding comp. I remember him saying to me "Phil, tense your delts [shoulders] harder!", and thinking to myself, "I am bloody tensing them!". I wasn't, though, and this is most likely why my shoulders don't grow overly well. The same is true of my legs. The left thigh I can barely flex, while the right one literally "pops" into action. Can you guess which leg is half an inch smaller? Yep, the left. It was posing lessons that made me realise I had some work to do on my "activation".

Activation exercises are used to practice flexing these less-than-responsive muscles if they are poor; and then, once they have improved, you can still use them to warm up a certain muscle. You'll often find that once you have some blood into the target muscle and a slight pump, it becomes easier to engage these muscles in your main movements. Using my shoulders as an example, I may do a few side raises and front raises prior to doing my main heavy shoulder presses. The key is to get them fired up but to not overly fatigue them. You don't want to ruin your chances of improving on your main lifts. For that reason, then, I tend to do just three to four sets of 12-15 reps with a very light weight, literally focusing on the muscle and flexing it on every rep until I feel like the muscle is connected to my brain better. It's then that I move onto my first exercise of the session. I personally only do this on the areas of the body I'm struggling with, as I've already discussed.

Key points -

- Activation exercises are used to practice or remember how to flex certain muscle groups.
- Although this isn't always the case, it is commonly the muscles that contribute to poor posture that will be affected, such as the muscles of the back, bum, and hips.
- These exercises can precede the main exercise of a muscle group, but be careful not to overly fatigue the muscle. A good example would be hamstring curls to engage the back of the thigh before going to do some squats.
- Only do three to four very light sets with really light weight. The main focus should be that you feel the muscle you are trying to target. Bear in mind that those muscles will often be fairly weak.

The cool-down

The cool-down is the phase that begins your recovery from an intense training session. The goal of the cool-down is to gently allow your body to transition from the intense exercise to being ready to safely leave the gym. For resistance training, you can use a cardiovascular machine, like a bike or treadmill, to warm the whole body back up. There are a couple of good reasons to do this.

Blood pooling

Doing a general whole-body movement will allow your blood to be moved around the body. When you perform resistance training, contractions from performing the exercises "pump" blood into the working muscles as you train. However, once you stop doing those exercises, you "switch off" that pump, and the blood can get trapped in the muscles you were working. This "pooling" of the blood can lead to you feeling faint or dizzy due to changes in blood pressure. It can be pretty uncomfortable, as well. The easy fix will be to get back on a bike or cross trainer for 5-10 minutes, at a low level, and gently move. The intensity needs to be low – this is not a time to try and burn off a few more calories. I know how people's minds work!

Post-training stretching

After training is a great to time to spend some time to stretch. Once you've rewarmed your body, you are ready to do some flexibility work. Similar to how I've explained how to stretch pre-training, doing it post-training would be the same. Holding stretches for 30-60 seconds and repeating that a couple of times will really help.

Contrary to what many people believe, the research doesn't really support that doing a cool-down after training will reduce the amount of soreness you'll experience. This was tested in normal active adults (Olsen et al., 2012) as well as professional Spanish football players (Rey et al., 2012 and Rey et al., 2012), and no differences were observed between those who did a cool down and those who practically just stopped exercising. However, that doesn't mean it's not worth doing. It just means that if you are pressed for time and need to get out of the gym in time for a meeting or to finish up some work at the office, you don't need to be concerned. Stretching can be done at other times of the day, as I said earlier. Do it after a warm bath, or walking to the shop, if you want. It's probably worth the majority of you saving 10-15 minutes to allow time to get your bodies warm, move the blood away from the working muscles, and get some light stretching done.

Cardiovascular training – "How much cardio shall I do?"

Cardiovascular training, aka "cardio", is something that, unfortunately, will need to be in most people's plans at some point. Cardio is basically any activity that raises your heart rate and burns calories. I'll always remember my lecturer at uni saying, "I wear my heart rate monitor in bed to make sure I'm working hard enough during sex". An odd admission, and we never did find out if he was telling the truth or not. Nevertheless, sex could definitely be classed as cardio – as long as you can last more than three minutes, of course. I won't insult you by spending too much time explaining the health benefits of regular cardio, but benefits do include:

• Reduced blood pressure
• Reduced risk of cardiovascular diseases
• Reduced risk of cancer
• Reduced risk of diabetes

- Reduction in bad cholesterol (LDL), with an increase in good (HDL) cholesterol

The NHS says that you only need to perform 150 minutes per week of moderate intensity activity, such as gardening, walking, and riding a bike, to get these benefits (Nhs.uk, 2015). For many of you, this will still be above what you regularly do. For the rest of this chapter, I'm going to discuss cardio with getting you into the best shape of your lives in mind. We know exercise is "healthy".

We have already discussed that the main driver for fat loss is ensuring that you are consistently in a calorie deficit. It's our daily energy balance that we must be concerned about. We can therefore affect fat loss by doing more activity or cardio. Cardio training usually goes into two main categories:

1. Steady state (SS) or aerobic training
2. High intensity interval training (HIIT)

Each one differs in intensity – in other words, how hard you work – and this is determined by your heart rate (HR) during the activity. The heart rate you need to work at for each category of cardio is calculated as a percentage of your "estimated maximum heart rate". Before we look at the different categories individually, let's look at how these percentages are calculated.

Your estimated maximum heart rate is based on your age, and is calculated as such:

220 - age = maximum heart rate

This means that if you are 45 years old, your maximum heart rate is 175 beats per minute (BPM). Each category of cardio will therefore have you working at a certain percentage of that estimated max heart rate. Simple. It's worth mentioning that the obvious flaw in this calculation is that it's entirely based on your age. It doesn't consider sex, exercise history, or even medical history, and therefore it would be best to use these recommendations as a good estimate or start point. For example, when I first left uni, I taught group cycling classes (often called spinning), and one of the participants was a guy who was a keen cyclist in his late 60's. This would have given him an estimated max heart rate of no more than 151, yet he routinely hit heart rates in the sprint sections of nearer 190! No, he didn't keel over halfway through the class. He was just very fit, slim, and had been training like that for the best part of 40-odd years. Is there a risk as you get older? Potentially, but that would be something I would suggest you discuss with your doctor should you be concerned. My point is that if you go over that "estimated max heart rate" and feel fine, it is not something to be alarmed about.

Steady state cardio

Usually referred to as "LISS", which stands for low intensity steady state, or "MISS", which is the same, just that the "M" stands for moderate, steady state cardio can simply be defined as any training session that is done over a prolonged period of time (usually 20-60 minutes in the context of the gym), with a fairly consistent heart rate maintained throughout. The British Heart Foundation recommends that this be done at around 50-70% of your max heart rate. For most people, though, a heart rate of 130-150 is reasonable, although as we have discussed already, it could be higher or lower depending on the individual.

If your first thought was that of someone doing a slow jog, or using an elliptical trainer staring at the clock, counting down the seconds, then you're on the right track. A good way to know that you're in the right heart rate training zone is that you should be working up a sweat, be breathing heavy, yet be able to hold a conversation fairly easily.

I'd like to provide you with some pros and cons of this method of cardio, to help you choose which type to do.

Steady state cardio pros:

1. It's very easy for the beginner, as the intensity isn't overwhelmingly hard.

2. Due to the intensity being low, it doesn't overly stress the body, and this makes it easy to recover from. Therefore, steady state cardio can be done fairly frequently throughout the week, allowing for more calories to be burned.

3. There are plenty of options that are low impact on the joints, making it great for someone who is slightly older or has injuries to consider. Swimming, cycling, and elliptical training are all far better choices than running (especially outside) if you need to be careful.

Steady state cardio cons:

1. It can be boring. As someone who did two 60-minute sessions a day, 6 days a week, for 7 weeks (the equivalent of 3.5 days!), I can attest to it becoming pretty dull. This can make it difficult to stay motivated. This will often be even worse if you are exercising indoors. For some, getting out of the house might be a better option.

For example, one of my clients lives in a rural part of Ireland, and he loves cycling the hills. For him, cardio (until the last month of his diet) was actually a pleasure.

2. Something that is very apparent is that the majority of people massively overestimate how many calories they actually burn during a steady state cardio session. I've had clients tell me that they had used over 1000 calories in a 45-minute session because the treadmill said so. I never put much weight into those readings, and the real danger here is that this information can often lead to people believing they can eat more food; or worse, that they deserve more food. I've heard so many people in my time in the fitness industry state that they go to the gym to be able to "eat what they want".

3. It can be very time-consuming. Most of my clients don't have time to do hour-long cardio sessions on top of their weight training. They simply don't have the time to commit to it. This is certainly something to consider. As you adapt to your plan, the only option with steady state cardio is to do more time.

4. Steady state cardio at higher intensities can be hard to recover from, especially while training with weights and restricting your body of calories – so doing high amounts of steady state cardio at higher intensities can ultimately lead to a loss of muscle and strength. *This is the exact opposite of what you want!* It's a bit of a cliché, but when was the last time you saw a marathon runner with decent shape and muscle? Not a look guys often choose to have.

5. Your body doesn't continue to burn calories after the session is finished, unlike high intensity cardio. This is something we'll discuss soon.

High-intensity interval training (HIIT)

High-intensity interval training – or "HIIT", as you'll usually see it called – is a form of training that has intervals of very intense exercise broken up by intervals of very easy exercise. This can then be repeated several times. The "work" interval commonly leads to heart rates of around 80-95% of a person's estimated max heart rate. This makes HIIT, quite frankly, horrible to perform. A common example would be:

1. Treadmill sprint - run as fast as possible for 30 seconds
2. Treadmill walk - slowly walk and recover for 90 seconds
3. Repeat 5-7 times in total

Due to the high intensity of those sprint phases, they will need to be very short in time, usually 10-30 seconds (although you'll often see people do intervals up to 60 seconds). Any longer, and it's impossible to maintain the high intensity needed. The rest periods then have to be very easy to allow for enough recovery to be able to maintain the high efforts required in the hard intervals. Here, you could rest completely or move slowly. A good recovery will be 60-120 seconds.

HIIT pros

1. It's much more time efficient than steady state cardio and this makes it a great option for those of you reading this. I rarely have people do more than 10 minutes of HIIT, and with a five-minute warm-up and a five-minute cool-down, this makes the whole session only 20 minutes in

total. It's much less of an ask for busy guys compared to 40-60 minutes of steady state training.

2. Even though you don't burn as many calories on a minute-to-minute basis during the session, your body will continue to burn calories after the session is over. This is due to something referred to as "excess post-exercise oxygen consumption", or EPOC. This means that even once you're back home relaxing, you're still getting the benefits. Not bad, right?

3. Some people will find it more bearable, because time doesn't seem to drag as much. I've heard people say this on many occasions, and I'm inclined to agree. This is due to the intensity of HIIT. It's pretty hard to worry about "clock watching" due to boredom when you're at the brink of passing out.

4. HIIT training such as sprinting has actually lead to some increases in muscle mass (Naimo et al., 2014), whereas lower intensity cardio would (in extreme cases) be more associated with muscle loss.

HIIT cons

1. Firstly, it's downright painful, or it should be if you work at the correct intensity. This makes it pretty much a no-no for beginners. I remember, stupidly, making my poor mum do several "life-threatening" intervals in my first year as a trainer, and I'm pretty sure she hasn't been back to a gym since. That was over 10 years ago! Whoops.

2. There is a definite increased risk of hurting yourself. A client of mine once tripped doing a fast sprint on the treadmill and practically got launched off the back of it. She was fine, fortunately. Unfortunately, the CCTV caught the whole thing on camera, and so we proceeded to record it and show the world. She did see the funny side of it. Eventually.

3. HIIT training is painful. End of. Oh, did I already mention this? Believe me, it bears repeating. The "burn" your muscles will experience is excruciating, and if you've done the session properly, you'll most likely end up on the floor in a pool of sweat wondering if you're going to puke or die. Now, the issue is that many people will not have the mental strength to push to these levels; therefore, the benefits are lost by them half-assing it. This definitely has to be considered before you choose to do some HIIT training.

4. Due to the high intensities needed, HIIT will take longer to recover from. In fact, if someone is doing HIIT correctly, I see those sessions almost like extra resistance training sessions, and therefore you must be careful with how many HIIT sessions you add to your programme. Yes, they will aid with fat loss, but if they overly hinder your recovery from your resistance training, then you run the risk of reducing your performance at your next session. This could make it more difficult to maintain muscle size and strength during the diet.

How to use cardio correctly for fat loss

If you're reading this and aren't currently exercising and haven't exercised in a long time, then I would advise you guys to begin with doing steady state training. This will be an easier way to get the ball rolling with training and improving your fitness, while burning calories for the reasons I addressed in the pros and cons. I'm not a fan of starting people with a lot of cardio to begin with, anyway. In most cases, those who aren't currently training, sit on their arses most of the time, and eat a crappy diet will easily lose weight by first addressing their diet, lifting some weights and just moving more. This leaves cardio as a great "ace card" that can be used further down the line when it's actually needed.

When you do decide to add some cardio to your programme, be cautious and start small. You can always add more. I'll usually start clients with three sessions of around 20-30 minutes max. As you become fitter and better able to work at higher intensities, you'll actually burn more calories; therefore, you might not even need to increase the length of your cardio sessions at first. At some point, your body will become accustomed to the length and intensity of your cardio sessions, and you'll be required to add more to maintain a calorie deficit and ensure you continue to lose fat.

Personally, I wouldn't add more cardio until it is absolutely necessary. You don't have to add cardio every time you plateau. You can, of course, reduce your food intake. That is your call. One of my clients, Mark, hates cardio, and it really messes with his knees. He chose to do ZERO cardio (he does walk daily, though) and simply eat less. On the other hand, Tim decided to walk more, seeing as he lives and works in London. He's now averaging 14,000 steps per day – that's roughly seven miles! That's on top of his three to four resistance training sessions. I've barely changed his food intake in weeks. Two different options, yet both yield the same results. Choose the path that suits you more.

Those of you who have already been exercising and are already slightly fitter have the option to include some HIIT training. The main thing to remember is that HIIT sessions are hard to recover from, especially for your poor legs. If you are training legs hard two or three times a week (like you should be), then believe me, you won't get that far adding in two or three hard sprint sessions. This must be taken into consideration, as well as which days you choose to do HIIT sessions. I don't believe that most people need more than two HIIT sessions per week. For most, this will give you the benefits of fat loss without unnecessarily increasing the risk of overworking yourself. If you can get away with more, then that's great, and you'll have to assess that yourself by closely recording how you feel, how you recover, and how your strength is improving in the gym. If you need more cardio after that, then of course, this is where you can utilise some steady state cardio.

In the beginning, when the amount of cardio you're doing is low, I would recommend doing it on your rest days from resistance training. This allows for better recovery, and allows you to devote your full energy to whatever session you're doing. For example:

Monday – Weights
Tuesday – Cardio
Wednesday – Weights
Thursday – Rest
Friday – Weights
Saturday – Cardio
Sunday – Rest

As your cardio needs increase, you may sometimes need to have a cardio session and resistance training session on the same day. My preference would be to keep them separate. For example, you could do cardio in the morning before work, and then do some weights later in the day at lunch or after work. For some of you, this will not be feasible due to your workload and other commitments, and clients will often ask me when it's "best" to do their cardio – before or after the resistance training. The answer is that you should do cardio after resistance training, to save as much energy for lifting weights as possible. As a side note, do be careful doing things like sprints after a training your legs. They will be very fatigued, and this increases the chances of injury. You do not want to be the next person filmed crashing off the back of the treadmill, to be making the rounds on social media. A better option here would be a bike, for example.

Remember, nothing is set in stone with fat loss, and you should always be prepared to try something new, as things can change quickly. Bear in mind that cardio may not be going up, but calories can be coming down, and this will also affect your recovery. One of my clients, Jon, who I've featured in a previous chapter, was doing fine with four weight training sessions per week. His cardio was a mix of SS and HIIT, with 2 HIIT sessions of around 10 minutes. I remember one week, he just hit the wall. His calories were low because he was almost four months into his diet, very near the end, in fact. Business was busy and he was working longer hours, and so I decided to remove the HIIT cardio altogether and replace it with some SS instead. This worked great. His ability to recover from the weight training improved almost instantly, and so he felt much less sore during the week. His leg training also improved, and he still maintained very good weekly losses in weight.

The important take-home point is that your decision on whether or not to use HIIT or SS cardio is based on a number of variables, including what you enjoy, what you can recover from, how much spare time you have on a day-to-day basis, and how your resistance training programme is set up. Many articles will tell you that a certain style of cardio is "better" than the other, but those articles fail to consider the most important part of the equation: you. A recent study actually showed no difference between doing steady state and high intensity interval training on fat loss (Keating et al., 2017). This is something I've noticed from my own training and working with hundreds of clients.

Non-exercise activity thermogenesis: "Why are you using the lifts?!"

Non-exercise activity thermogenesis (NEAT for short) refers to the energy you use on a daily basis that isn't from formal exercise. Researchers define it like so:

"NEAT is the thermogenesis that accompanies physical activities other than volitional exercise, such as the activities of daily living, fidgeting, spontaneous muscle contraction, and maintaining posture when not recumbent or eating." (Levine, 2002)

Good examples are:

- Walking more by ditching the car
- Gardening/mowing the lawn
- Sex (if you put in the work and can last long enough…)
- Cleaning the house
- Taking the stairs instead of the lift

Remember that you're trying to create a calorie deficit by restricting calorie intake from food and drinks and increasing energy expenditure through activity, in order to burn body fat. Most guys simply don't consider that their actions on a day-to-day basis can either help or hinder their progress. Consider the difference between someone who is doing three gym sessions per week and who works 10 hours on a building site, to the guy who trains three times a week and sits at the desk for 10 hours per day. The builder is going to burn a ton more calories per day and this should make dieting far easier for him. Chances are that the builder won't ever need to diet in the first place – unless his career builds and he ends up behind a desk.

If you're overweight and have been sedentary for many years, then in all likelihood, you're going to have poor habits when it comes to simply moving. You're probably more likely to drive to the shop, not walk. If there is the choice between the stairs and a lift, you'll stand there waiting for the lift. I remember one time I came back from London on the train. It was about 6pm, and therefore the train was rammed. Upon arrival at Reading, I made my way to the stairs and proceeded to climb them. I suddenly realised I was the only one climbing them, and so I looked back at the train to see the rest of the passengers, every single one, <u>queuing</u> for the escalator. I remember wondering how those people could be lazy enough to waste so much of their time in situations like that, as well as just taking their health for granted. It's worth noting, because people who move less in general are going to find weight management more difficult than those like me, who use the stairs.

It's important that I cover this. By definition, dieting means you're providing your body with less calories than it needs, and this can lead to increased fatigue and lower energy levels, which will affect your levels of NEAT. This is an extreme example, but from my own experience, I can say that when I dieted for my bodybuilding competition, by the time I was around 20 weeks into the diet (8 weeks away from the event), I was literally struggling to even do my training. The gym where I train people doesn't have a car park, so we have to park about half a mile away – a six-minute walk at most. By the time I was close to my competition, I was having to take several mini breaks to get there, I was simply that tired. One time that walk took me nearly 20 minutes! The result of this had a drastic effect on my energy output each day. This is probably why I ended needing to spend two hours a day on an exercise machine.

What you need to try and do, the best you can, is maintain your daily NEAT throughout the duration of your diet. This can be done very simply in a number of ways. The easiest would be to track how many steps you take per day using a fitness watch or pedometer. Just so you know, the NHS recommends a daily step target of 10,000, although the average performed by most is just 3,000-4,000 (NHS, 2017). If every one of you just upped how much you walked each day, you'd easily improve your health and drop some fat. There are also apps that you can download to phones to track activity like cleaning, gardening, and shopping. Yes, not exactly things that excite us guys, but think of the bigger picture here.

You could also have things that you commit to doing on a daily basis, and stick to it regardless of how tired you are. For example, no matter how tired I became during my diet, without fail I'd still take my dogs for a walk every evening for 20-30 minutes. It was something that I simply wouldn't dare miss. It would be extremely selfish of me as a dog owner to not take them because I'm tired. That was some powerful accountability. Find something similar. Commit to taking your wife to that dance class she's been nagging about, play with the children or grandchildren, take some time to walk to get lunch instead of driving there. Consider helping out around the house, be it washing the dishes, putting away some laundry, or vacuuming. Not only are you being active, but the wife will be delighted, and with that extra free time and energy she now has, maybe you can even get some more – ahem – "cardio" in later in the evening. Do whatever it takes to keep you moving, and do so consistently!

Then simply track it. If your steps per day start to drop, use that information to correct it. If you have decided that you will walk to the shop every day for the newspaper, and then begin resorting to reading it online, give yourself a stern talking to and change it.

If you're one of those guys whose routine consists of waking up, driving to work, sitting at the desk, driving home, and then sitting on your arse, then you need to increase your movement from the very beginning. Do it. Not just for weight loss, but to begin forming a more active lifestyle that will benefit you for the rest of your life.

Chapter 5

The stuff you won't consider

Over the years, I've had tons of questions from guys asking for my advice on training, food intake, and supplements, but something I'm rarely asked is for help with actually dealing with making those lifestyle changes. There are many factors that will make essentially simple changes feel extremely difficult at times. The aim of this chapter is to prepare you for those challenges, and arm you with some solutions, so that you can keep making progress as intended.

Other people making it difficult – "MUM! I'm dieting!"

When you finally make that big decision to change your lifestyle and improve your health and fitness, there is good chance you'll begin to feel very alone. It's very likely that you'll be the only one in your family and your entire group of friends trying to make this change. This makes you a minority. Those around you begin to see you as different, and you'll experience some issues because of this.

I've witnessed many clients getting resistance from their partners, wives, family, and friends when attempting to improve their health and fitness. You would assume that your loved ones would be very supportive of you making the kinds of changes that not only benefit you, but them also. Sadly, the reality is that this isn't always the case. I've seen it time and time again, where the people closest to my clients have actively tried to sabotage their efforts to succeed. Examples of this are people deliberately offering (or teasing them with) foods that they know they're trying to avoid, making them feel bad for wanting to eat something different, and moaning about the amount of time they're spending at the gym, amongst many others.

I can only assume this is due to them feeling envious of the fact that someone close to them is doing something that they may wish they had the motivation to do. I also suspect that often, seeing someone make positive changes to their health and fitness makes those around them realise how badly they're doing. The person who is working on improving themselves is like a "reality check" mirror, always reminding that other person that they aren't reaching their potential. This reminds me of "crab mentality", or the "crab in a bucket" analogy, where if you were to put a group of crabs into a bucket, they could all easily escape; yet instead, any crab that attempts to climb out will get pulled back down by the rest of the crabs. This is why you shouldn't associate with people who don't share your goals, ambitions and positive attitude, as they will always try to keep you at their level. Many of you will experience an element of this at some point along the way.

In fact, one woman I trained many years ago was fairly overweight, and so was her husband. Regardless of her body shape, she was still very attractive – and I knew that once she had lost some weight, she would begin to turn a lot of heads. We've all seen women (and men) transform like that, especially nowadays with social media making it possible to see people's achievements from all over the world. After several months of dieting and training with me, she proved me right and looked amazing. The problem was that her husband chose to continue his normal way of life. The whole time he was negative, he would eat takeaways in front of her, and he'd tell her she was taking it too seriously. As my client gained more confidence and turned more and more heads, he became very insecure about himself. The knock-on effect, as you can probably guess, was that he became more and more clingy, paranoid, and, in her own words, "less attractive". Eventually, they broke up. This is probably a somewhat extreme example, yet it goes to show why some people will not like to see you improving yourself.

There will be some friends and family that just simply won't understand what you need to do to be successful, and as a result, they will do things that make dieting harder. Usually not in a spiteful or malicious way, though. For example, my mum, bless her, was a great example of this. When my girlfriend was dieting for her first bikini competition, on a daily basis, Mum would offer her things like biscuits, sweets, and wine. "I'm sure a little won't hurt", she would say. Something I bet you have all heard someone say at some point before. The problem is that those extra calories can hurt if you're not careful – even more so if you were to give in to every single person that offered you some food!

This scenario can put you in a bit of a tight spot. You'll want to simply say, "No thank you", and carry on with your diet, but you'll most likely also be concerned about offending people. Honestly, I can't remember ever having anyone take offence because I declined something they had offered me. However, I still recommend that you take the time to explain *why* you can't accept something they are offering. The good thing here is that if you do this, they'll often not ask you again out of respect for you and the importance of your goals.

For many guys, this will be an issue of discipline. Some of you might find it difficult to say no, and easily give in to the temptation of what's on offer. This is something you will definitely have to address. Learn to say, "No thanks". Get into the habit of doing so, and you will find that it will become easier and easier over time. We'll discuss something that will help with this in another chapter.

Social situations – "I feel weird doing this…"

Social situations, like dinners, parties, and business meetings also provide a time where sticking to healthier habits can be difficult. I find that many clients have concerns during these situations as it can feel awkward and even embarrassing for many ordering a "healthy" meal in front of friends, being the only one to skip dessert, telling people you're not drinking, and eating your own food brought from home. Doing these things always seems to stir up interest amongst the people you're with. You will probably get 'interrogated' with common questions like, "Why are YOU dieting?", "Why are you being boring?", and "Why do you go to the gym so much?". I can't remember a single client who hasn't, at some point during their time with me, mentioned this during one of their check-ins or Skype calls.

This is something you'll have to learn to deal with; and quite frankly, my best advice is to have a pair of balls big enough to be able to answer those questions with confidence and complete honesty. For me, it's very easy. I'm outspoken, confident, and to be honest, I don't mind offending people in situations like these.

This is the way I would deal with a stupid question:

Friend: "Phil, why do you need to go to the gym so much?"
Me: "Because it beats being lazy, out of shape, and feeling like shit…"

Simple and to the point. Of course, I don't expect many of you reading this to be so bold (or perhaps rude), but you will need to deal with these situations well. Some advice I'll offer you from experience is this: Be confident. Confidence is the one trait you'll need to possess from now on in order to get the best from this new lifestyle. Be confident that deep down in your heart, you are happy with your choice to make these new changes – no matter what anyone else thinks or says about you. It's YOUR life, and you can do with it as you please. If you never want to drink another beer again, want to swap the pub for the gym, or sit and eat homemade meals while everyone else is eating a curry, that is YOUR choice. If you're truly confident with those choices, truly believe in them, and above all else, are happy about them, then what others think about those choices will no longer matter to you – you simply won't fucking care.

This is a very powerful place to be. At this point, everyone else's opinions will no longer trouble you. You will find it much easier to deal with situations like this, because you won't feel unproductive emotions such as embarrassment and insecurity – especially when your mates take the piss out of you, which, if they are real mates, they will. Here's an example for you: I'm lazy, and I hate cooking. Therefore, for my fat intake, I often literally swig some olive oil from the bottle – it's pretty rank, but it's simple and time efficient. Do you know how many people look at me like I'm some kind of freak? Many. Do you know how much I care? Fuck all.

All I care about is getting my food right at that moment and continuing to take steps towards my goals. This is a mentality that I strongly recommend you strive for. It will serve you well in all walks of life.

Fitness in a business environment

I once had a conversation with my long-term client Paul. I asked him how he found sticking to his healthy lifestyle in a business environment. He told me that it doesn't bother him being seen to be choosing healthy foods, and that he was happier to have just one beer before switching back to water, even if everyone he was with carried on drinking alcohol. He explained that he never feels pressured to do as the others are doing just to "fit in" or not feel out of place. This, he said, was a stark contrast to how his partner thinks and acts in these situations. His partner, also successful in business, doesn't like the idea of standing out and being different. He feels that doing so might reflect poorly on him and could jeopardise the relationships he's trying to build. In other words, it might not help the business be successful. These are very different attitudes, and it's probably obvious which of the two is the healthiest (although that is just one variable to consider).

Many of you, too, will find it difficult to stay on track in these situations. In fact, I would bet that many of you would use them as an excuse to justify getting off-track. If you're someone who regularly meets new prospects and clients, has to travel and attend meetings, then you're going to not only need a plan that is flexible (which, having read this book, you will), but you're going to need to learn to feel confident and content about potentially standing out. Sure, you can have the odd beer, and the odd hotel fry up won't ruin your chances of success, but they will need to be far less frequent than you're used to.

Be prepared to be different and have some self-control.

The importance of "ticking all the boxes"

Many men, especially beginners, fail to appreciate the importance of consistently getting as much of this information right as possible. This is, however, vital if you want to continuously make progress.

Here, I'm referring to:

- Quality and consistency of your diet
- Sleep quality and a suitable number of hours (6-8 for most)
- Stress levels
- Water intake for hydration
- How you've structured your training throughout the week

Not so long ago, I was reminded of how essential this is. The time came to try a new personal best on one of my main exercises. After the previous time doing that lift, I felt really confident that it would go well. When I woke up the morning of that training session, I wasn't as confident. Not only did I not get that personal best (or PB), I was actually unable to lift the previous week's best. In fact, I was nearly 30kg from it! What was different? Well, going back to those variables above, I'd pretty much screwed them all up.

At the time, my mum was terminally ill. I won't dwell on that here, but it's a fact that needed to be stated to add some context to this example. The weekend prior to that awful training session, I'd been to visit her, and her health had really declined since the last time I'd seen her, just a couple of weeks before. The whole situation led to a sharp decline in the length and quality of my sleep, as I was getting up to help her in the night. I was under a great deal more stress, too, and I'll admit it was at that point in time when it began to take its toll.

Around that time, I also started suffering from tension migraines. I've never had them before, and for those of you who do suffer with them on a regular basis, I feel your pain. I'd been getting them every week or so, and I physically can't do anything, let alone train. As you can imagine, I wasn't really eating well either, certainly not how I'd usually eat. Basically, everything was pretty messed up around that time, and this all led up to that disgrace of a training session.

As a side note, if you're wondering why I still trained given those circumstances, then it's because exercise makes me feel better and allows me to deal with life events like this more easily. Many of you will witness this great benefit in the near future, I hope. My example is rather extreme, but every one of you will have things come up that make training harder. Businesses to run, children to look after, friends to help, etc. Do your best to manage those things, as they can and certainly will affect your results if you do not.

My main point is to remember that what you do in the days prior to training will certainly dictate how well you perform. If you're the person who doesn't meet calorie needs, doesn't sleep well, and forgets to stay hydrated – FIX those things before you worry about anything else. I lost one good session, that won't do any harm, but I guarantee that some of you will rarely be at your very best for the reasons I've stated. I've had clients turn up to train with me having had only coffee all day, who are hungover and exhausted, and they all had one thing in common – I sent them home.

Let this be a reminder that having good health and fitness is a process that needs to be applied very consistently if you want to really be your very best. It isn't something you can pick and choose to do when it suits you. Make it the focal point of your life. Write a diary for food and water, use an app to keep track of your sleep, etc., and if something doesn't feel right, fix it. I guarantee that everything will fall into place if you consistently get those (seemingly) small things right.

What to do with this information (if you want to succeed)

There you have it. Here is the result of eighteen-odd years of studying, being in the gym, working with people 1-2-1, and making every mistake I could have made, all in one place. The point of sharing this is that you can learn from those mistakes, avoid doing yet another "fad diet", stop believing all those nonsensical fitness "myths", and **finally** get some results – and importantly, as I've harped on about a million times already, be able to maintain them for a lifetime. Long-term success really is the "holy grail" of fitness.

The take-home message of this book is that in order for you to achieve your fitness goals, you must accept that there is more than one way to skin a cat. I know that's very cliché, but it's also very true. In other words, the diet and fitness programme that best helps you achieve your goals is the one that is objectively best for you – no matter what any article or professional with a "one-size-fits-all" approach tells you. Getting your head around this is crucial, because although most of you appear to be similar – in other words, 40+ year old men that run successful businesses, have families to look after, and a social life to juggle – this doesn't mean that your fitness programme will look anything like anyone else's.

There will be differences in:

- What your goals are and the reasons for them
- What injuries you have that will affect the training programme
- How much exercise time you have on a regular basis
- What foods you like, dislike and are even intolerant to
- Whether you can eat in the office or are you someone who travels a lot
- How well you cope with stress
- How well you sleep and how much sleep you need

I could go on and on.

For example, some of you may spend much of your time in the office, meaning you can eat homemade meals whenever you want very simply. On the other hand, some of you will be travelling a lot, meaning that you frequently will have to eat in hotels, restaurants and at airports. Clearly, then, a "cookie cutter" approach would no doubt increase the chances of failure for some of you. If I've got this book right, then the idea that you can be fairly flexible with your approach to improving your fitness and health should be well ingrained. By this point, you should be ready to use this book to create a plan that fits your needs and lifestyle – contrary to the more common approach of trying to force your lifestyle and needs to fit into a plan, like some sort of fitness contortionist.

The key to this type of approach is still understanding that there are "parameters of best practice"; certain ways in which fitness can not only bring you success, but be sustainable enough for your needs and lifestyle to bring you long-term success. I've gone on and on about how poor the stats are of people losing weight and maintaining weight loss long-term, so you don't need me to say it again; but fuck, it I will. The most important aspect of any diet or fitness plan is your ability to adhere to it, day in, day out, year in, year out. Anyone can drop some weight fast when something important like a holiday or wedding is coming up, but the methods used to achieve that goal are often gruelling and short-sighted. I, therefore, challenge you to see your fitness and health as something you will make a long-term priority.

For that, you need something you can follow long-term. I remember a client of mine who couldn't maintain weight loss, no matter what I did. She would lose several pounds, then put it back on. This cycle continued for literally years. I did everything I could to keep her on track, but I just couldn't. She just couldn't see the bigger picture. She obsessed over the little details before she could get the most important things right. One day, at the end of one of her sessions she said to me, "How much weight should I be losing each week? Should I be losing more?", to which I replied, "Don't focus on how much weight you can lose each week, but on how many weeks you can lose weight".

That one statement pretty much sums up what every one of you should be focusing on: consistency. My client Jenny lost ~54kg (8.5 stone!), but at a much slower rate than you'd predict it "could" be lost. Sure, it was slower, but the main thing was that over that time, she developed a lifestyle that was sustainable. At the end of the day, we got the job done, and she's kept the weight off. Importantly, she doesn't hate the way in which we went about it. Training is fun, she has some great goals to work towards, and she's learnt that if you follow a few rules and keep yourself accountable, you can keep the weight off, feel great, and still eat and drink what the hell you want at times. *We found the perfect balance of success, consistency, and being happy to keep doing the work.*

That was the goal of this book: to show you that there are options in almost every aspect of diet and fitness that can be manipulated to fit into your lifestyle. Whether you're choosing to train three times instead of five, or you want to eat four larger meals rather than seven smaller meals, the information in this book allows you to make those choices while keeping you within the boundaries that both experience and science shows to be acceptable for getting results.

Lastly, though, and this is important, there is a huge difference between knowing what to do and actually doing it. There will be many of you who read this, and then simply put it on the shelf to collect dust with the rest of your "how-to" collection. That's the way it is. I can't change that, but I will still say that despite the fact I've tried my hardest to provide you with all the information needed to make dieting easier than you've ever done it before, that doesn't mean that it won't take hard work, discipline, and some sacrifices. If you're serious about losing your "business bod", then be prepared to make some changes and get outside of your comfort zone.

Think of it like your business. Would it be successful if you just hoped all would be okay, without taking any risks, making any sacrifices, or putting in any effort? Of course not! You had to put the work in. You had days that were frustrating, hard work, and made you want to quit. Nonetheless, you persevered and made it successful. Take that attitude with how you deal with improving your fitness, and believe me, there will be no stopping you.

Good luck with it all. I really hope this book was the catalyst needed to get you ready to change your life forever. Remember to go to www.philagostino.co.uk/bonus and use all the free resources that will further educate you and aid you with your transformation.

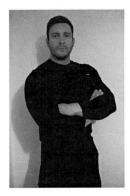

Phil Agostino

References

Acheson, K. (1993). Influence of autonomic nervous system on nutrient-induced thermogenesis in humans. Nutrition, 9, pp.373-80.

Agarwal, K., Tripathi, C., Agarwal, B. and Saluja, S. (2011). Efficacy of turmeric (curcumin) in pain and post-operative fatigue after laparoscopic cholecystectomy: a double-blind, randomized placebo-controlled study. Surgical Endoscopy, 25(12), pp.3805-3810.

Aragon, A. (2008). Nutrient Timing, Part 1: Fat. Alan Aragon's Research Review (AARR), [online] January, pp.2-5. Available at: https://alanaragon.com [Accessed 7 Feb. 2017].

Aragon, A. (2008). Nutrient Timing, Part 2: Pre- & During Exercise Carboyhydrate & Protein. Alan Aragon's Research Review, [online] pp.2-8. Available at: https://alanaragon.com/subscribers-area/ [Accessed 9 Apr. 2017].

Astrup, A. (2005). 'The satiating power of protein - a key

to obesity prevention?'. American Journal of Clinical Nutrition, [online] 82(1), pp.1-2. Available at: http://ajcn.nutrition.org/content/82/1/1.full.pdf+html [Accessed 6 Nov. 2016].

Bellisle, F., McDevitt, R. and Prentice, A. (1997). Meal frequency and energy balance. British Journal of Nutrition, [online] 77(S1), p.S57. Available at: https://www.cambridge.org/core/services/aop-cambridge-core/content/view/S0007114597000093 [Accessed 27 Nov. 2016].

Beulens, J., Bots, M., Atsma, F., Bartelink, M., Prokop, M., Geleijnse, J., Witteman, J., Grobbee, D. and van der Schouw, Y. (2009). High dietary menaquinone intake is associated with reduced coronary calcification. Atherosclerosis, [online] 203(2), pp.489-493. Available at: https://www.researchgate.net/publication/23189487_High_dietary_menaquinone_intake_is_associated_with_reduced_coronary_calcification [Accessed 6 Mar. 2017].

Biesalski, H. (2002). Meat and cancer: meat as a component of a healthy diet. European Journal of Clinical Nutrition, [online] 56(s1), pp.S2-S11. Available at: https://www.ncbi.nlm.nih.gov/pubmed/11965516 [Accessed 1 Jun. 2017].

Biolo, G., Williams, B., Fleming, R. and Wolfe, R. (1999). Insulin action on muscle protein kinetics and amino acid transport during recovery after resistance exercise. Diabetes, 48(5), pp.949-57.

Burke, L. (2008). Caffeine and sports performance. Applied Physiology, Nutrition, and Metabolism, [online] 33(6), pp.1319-1334. Available at: https://www.researchgate.net/publication/23669680_Caffeine_and_sport_performance

[Accessed 6 Mar. 2017].

Campbell, B., Kreider, R., Ziegenfuss, T., La Bounty, P., Roberts, M., Burke, D., Landis, J., Lopez, H. and Antonio, J. (2007). International Society of Sports Nutrition position stand: protein and exercise. Journal of the International Society of Sports Nutrition, [online] 4(1), p.8. Available at: https://jissn.biomedcentral.com/articles/10.1186/1550-2783-4-8 [Accessed 5 Aug. 2017].

Cannell, J. (2013). Vitamin D Council | Why does the Vitamin D Council recommend 5,000 IU/day?. [online] Vitamindcouncil.org. Available at: https://www.vitamindcouncil.org/why-does-the-vitamin-d-council-recommend-5000-iu-day/ [Accessed 24 Feb. 2017].

Chainani-Wu, N. (2003). Safety and Anti-Inflammatory Activity of Curcumin: A Component of Tumeric (Curcuma longa). The Journal of Alternative and Complementary Medicine, [online] 9(1), pp.161-168. Available at: http://www.olivamine.com/sites/default/files/research/Curcumin-Safety.pdf [Accessed 7 Jan. 2017].

Chow, L. (2006). Mechanism of insulin's anabolic effect on muscle: measurements of muscle protein synthesis and breakdown using aminoacyl-tRNA and other surrogate measures. AJP: Endocrinology and Metabolism, [online] 291(4), pp.E729-E736. Available at: http://ajpendo.physiology.org/content/291/4/E729 [Accessed 5 May 2017].

Chowdhury, R., Warnakula, S., Kunutsor, S., Crowe, F., Ward, H., Johnson, L., Franco, O., Butterworth, A., Forouhi, N., Thompson, S., Khaw, K., Mozaffarian, D.,

Danesh, J. and Di Angelantonio, E. (2014). Association of Dietary, Circulating, and Supplement Fatty Acids With Coronary Risk. Annals of Internal Medicine, [online] 160(6), pp.398-406. Available at: https://www.ncbi.nlm.nih.gov/pubmed/24723079 [Accessed 6 May 2017].

ChwalbiÃ±ska-Moneta, L. (2003). Effect of creatine supplementation on aerobic performance and anaerobic capacity in elite rowers in the course of endurance training. International Journal of Sport Nutrition and Exercise Metabolism, [online] 13(2), pp.173-83. Available at: https://www.ncbi.nlm.nih.gov/pubmed/12945828 [Accessed 2 Feb. 2017].

Davoodi, S., Ajami, M., Ayatollahi, S., Dowlatshahi, K., Javedan, G. and Pazoki-Toroud, H. (2014). Calorie Shifting Diet Versus Calorie Restriction Diet: A Comparative Clinical Trial Study. International journal of preventive medicine, [online] 5(4), pp.447â€"456. Available at: http://International journal of preventive medicine [Accessed 25 Sep. 2016].

Dhurandhar, E., Dawson, J., Alcorn, A., Larsen, L., Thomas, E., Cardel, M., Bourland, A., Astrup, A., St-Onge, M., Hill, J., Apovian, C., Shikany, J. and Allison, D. (2014). The effectiveness of breakfast recommendations on weight loss: a randomized controlled trial. American Journal of Clinical Nutrition, [online] 100(2), pp.507-513. Available at: https://www.ncbi.nlm.nih.gov/pmc/articles/PMC4095657/ [Accessed 26 Oct. 2016].

DiSilvestro, R., Joseph, E., Zhao, S. and Bomser, J. (2012). Diverse effects of a low dose supplement of lipidated curcumin in healthy middle aged people. Nutrition Journal, [online] 11(79). Available at: https://nutritionj.biomedcentral.com/articles/10.1186/1475-2891-11-79 [Accessed 12 Jul. 2017].

Dorgan, J., Judd, J., Longcope, C., Brown, C., Schatzkin, A., Clevidence, B., Campbell, W., Nair, P., Franz, C., Kahle, L. and Taylor, P. (1996). Effects of dietary fat and fiber on plasma and urine androgens and estrogens in men: a controlled feeding study. The American Journal of Clinical Nutrition, [online] 64(6), pp.850-5. Available at: http://ajcn.nutrition.org/content/64/6/850.abstract [Accessed 3 Oct. 2016].
En.wikipedia.org. (2017). 5 Whys. [online] Available at: https://en.wikipedia.org/wiki/5_Whys [Accessed 3 Jul. 2017].

Esmaily, H., Sahebkar, A., Iranshahi, M., Ganjali, S., Mohammadi, A., Ferns, G. and Ghayour-Mobarhan, M. (2015). An investigation of the effects of curcumin on anxiety and depression in obese individuals: A randomized controlled trial. Chinese Journal of Integrative Medicine, [online] 21(5), pp.332-338. Available at: https://link.springer.com/article/10.1007/s11655-015-2160-z [Accessed 2 Jan. 2017].

Fildes, A., Charlton, J., Rudisill, C., Littlejohns, P., Prevost, A. and Gulliford, M. (2015). Probability of an Obese Person Attaining Normal Body Weight: Cohort Study Using Electronic Health Records. American Journal of Public Health, [online] 105(9), pp.e54-e59. Available at: http://ajph.aphapublications.org/doi/full/10.2105/AJPH.2015.302773 [Accessed 28 Feb. 2017].

Frank, K., Patel, K., Lopez, G. and Willis, B. (2017). Fish Oil Research Analysis. [online] Examine.com. Available at: https://examine.com/supplements/fish-oil/ [Accessed 27

Feb. 2017].

Frank, K., Patel, K., Lopez, G. and Willis, B. (2017). Vitamin K Research Analysis. [online] Examine.com. Available at: https://examine.com/supplements/vitamin-k/ [Accessed 4 Mar. 2017].

Frank, K., Patel, K., Lopez, G. and Willis, B. (2017). Curcumin Research Analysis. [online] Examine.com. Available at: https://examine.com/supplements/curcumin/ [Accessed 2 Jan. 2017].

Frank, K., Patel, K., Lopez, G. and Willis, B. (2017). Magnesium Research Analysis. [online] Examine.com. Available at: https://examine.com/supplements/Magnesium/ [Accessed 3 Jan. 2017].

Geleijnse, J., Vermeer, C., Grobbee, D., Schurgers, L., Knapen, M., van der Meer, I., Hofman, A. and Witteman, J. (2004). Dietary Intake of Menaquinone Is Associated with a Reduced Risk of Coronary Heart Disease: The Rotterdam Study. Journal of Nutrition, [online] 134(11), pp.3100-5. Available at: http://jn.nutrition.org/content/134/11/3100.long [Accessed 7 Mar. 2017].

Goldstein, E., Ziegenfuss, T., Kalman, D., Kreider, R., Campbell, B., Wilborn, C., Taylor, L., Willoughby, D., Stout, J., Graves, B., Wildman, R., Ivy, J., Spano, M., Smith, A. and Antonio, J. (2010). International society of sports nutrition position stand: caffeine and performance. Journal of the International Society of Sports Nutrition, [online] 7(1), p.5. Available at: https://jissn.biomedcentral.com/articles/10.1186/1550-2783-7-5 [Accessed 8 Mar. 2017].

Gorham, E., Garland, C., Garland, F., Grant, W., Mohr, S., Lipkin, M., Newmark, H., Giovannucci, E., Wei, M. and Holick, M. (2007). Optimal Vitamin D Status for Colorectal Cancer Prevention. American Journal of Preventive Medicine, [online] 32(3), pp.210-216. Available at: http://www.direct-ms.org/sites/default/files/ColonMetaAnalysisPaper.pdf [Accessed 22 Feb. 2017].

Gov.uk. (2017). Modern life responsible for â€˜worryingâ€™ health in middle aged - GOV.UK. [online] Available at: https://www.gov.uk/government/news/modern-life-responsible-for-worrying-health-in-middle-aged [Accessed 3 Jul. 2017].

Grandjean, A., Reimers, K., Bannick, K. and Haven, M. (2000). The Effect of Caffeinated, Non-Caffeinated, Caloric and Non-Caloric Beverages on Hydration. Journal of the American College of Nutrition, [online] 19(5), pp.591-600. Available at: https://pdfs.semanticscholar.org/ad0d/f71c608fc71225746d550b42e010fbfe4fcc.pdf [Accessed 30 Aug. 2016].

Graudal, N., JÃ¼rgens, G., Baslund, B. and Alderman, M. (2014). Compared With Usual Sodium Intake, Low- and Excessive-Sodium Diets Are Associated With Increased Mortality: A Meta-Analysis. American Journal of Hypertension, [online] 27(9), pp.1129-1137. Available at: https://oup.silverchair-cdn.com/oup/backfile/Content_public/Journal/ajh/27/9/10.1093_ajh_hpu028/7/hpu028.pdf?Expires=1499951331&Signature=CB58h3tdVkV5lv-SGvNsQBljNMeUZhIF1e2rqZqq3Xj7mL8rTTVXlYXAIkupn78PIIlPbZNtkVlRmYBJwSTNBcJTbC-hryvqrDe0IRi70GCTdZrimDLv7aiKwig1q-bbLd6Arss4sm-

rlsQxmAS3RE2QPTvyioVdJlE5ZWSwMGvp7FwyL-
7gxXoUo~Rdf5dtqHmMiJixhEnfFuIH7UkuTknX-
7VU1OAVgwwRl3UVk9e3AVy7WBoEmaZAMwSFjP-
pA5GmwfesUYULJ~9Ij-QtdfD-YSNm8UbcZBwOw-
PUzWvQ-x~QF5rZ6IK1tAsK4DeFGDQ9G6XBgj4bX-
w7TzZ47gqZliaA__&Key-Pair-Id=APKAIUCZBI-
A4LVPAVW3Q [Accessed 28 Feb. 2017].

Ha, S. (2014). Dietary Salt Intake and Hypertension. Electrolytes & Blood Pressure, [online] 12(1), p.7. Available at:
https://www.ncbi.nlm.nih.gov/pmc/articles/PMC4105387/
[Accessed 28 Mar. 2017].

HämäläInen, E., Adlercreutz, H., Puska, P. and Piet-
inen, P. (1983). Decrease of serum total and free testosterone
during a low-fat high-fibre diet. Journal of Steroid Biochem-
istry, [online] 18(3), pp.369-370. Available at: https://www.
ncbi.nlm.nih.gov/pubmed/6298507 [Accessed 2 Jun. 2017].

Hanai, H., Iida, T., Takeuchi, K., Watanabe, F., Maruyama,
Y., Andoh, A., Tsujikawa, T., Fujiyama, Y., Mitsuyama, K.,
Sata, M., Yamada, M., Iwaoka, Y., Kanke, K., Hiraishi, H.,
Hirayama, K., Arai, H., Yoshii, S., Uchijima, M., Nagata,
T. and Koide, Y. (2006). Curcumin Maintenance Therapy for Ulcerative Colitis: Randomized, Multicenter, Double-Blind, Placebo-Controlled Trial. Clinical Gastroenterol-
ogy and Hepatology, [online] 4(12), pp.1502-1506. Available
at: https://www.researchgate.net/publication/6696893_Cur-
cumin_Maintenance_Therapy_for_Ulcerative_Colitis_Ran-
domized_Multicenter_Double-Blind_Placebo-Controlled_
Trial [Accessed 3 Jan. 2017].

Harcombe, Z., Baker, J., DiNicolantonio, J., Grace, F. and Davies, B. (2016). Evidence from randomised controlled trials does not support current dietary fat guidelines: a systematic review and meta-analysis. Open Heart, [online] 3(2), p.e000409. Available at: http://openheart.bmj.com/content/2/1/e000196 [Accessed 7 Dec. 2016].

He, F. and MacGregor, G. (2007). Salt, blood pressure and cardiovascular disease. Current Opinion in Cardiology, 22(4), pp.298-305.

Helms, E., Zinn, C., Rowlands, D. and Brown, S. (2014). A Systematic Review of Dietary Protein during Caloric Restriction in Resistance Trained Lean Athletes: A Case for Higher Intakes. International Journal of Sport Nutrition and Exercise Metabolism, [online] 24(2), pp.127-138. Available at: https://www.researchgate.net/profile/Scott_Brown12/publication/257350851_A_Systematic_Review_of_Dietary_Protein_During_Caloric_Restriction_in_Resistance_Trained_Lean_Athletes_A_Case_for_Higher_Intakes/links/0f31753bc6ad63f47f000000.pdf [Accessed 19 Sep. 2016].

Hill, M. (2002). Meat, cancer and dietary advice to the public. European Journal of Clinical Nutrition, [online] 56(s1), pp.S36-S41. Available at: https://www.ncbi.nlm.nih.gov/pubmed/11965521 [Accessed 1 May 2017].

Hill, M. (2002). Meat, cancer and dietary advice to the public. European Journal of Clinical Nutrition, [online] 56(s1), pp.S36-S41. Available at: https://www.nature.com/ejcn/journal/v56/n1s/pdf/1601352a.pdf?origin=ppub [Accessed 4 Jul. 2017].

Hussein, N., Ah-Sing, E., Wilkinson, P., Leach, C., Griffin, B. and Millward, D. (2004). Long-chain conversion of [13C]linoleic acid and Î±-linolenic acid in response to marked changes in their dietary intake in men. Journal of Lipid Research, [online] 46(2), pp.269-280. Available at: http://www.jlr.org/content/46/2/269.full [Accessed 28 Feb. 2017].

Johnston, C., Tjonn, S., Swan, P. and White, A. (2017).

Johnston, C., Tjonn, S., Swan, P., White, A., Hutchins, H. and Sears, B. (2006). Ketogenic low-carbohydrate diets have no metabolic advantage over nonketogenic low-carbohydrate diets. The American Journal of Clinical Nutrition, [online] 83(5), pp.1055-61. Available at: http://ajcn.nutrition.org/content/83/5/1055.full.pdf [Accessed 25 Jan. 2017].

Keating, S., Johnson, N., Mielke, G. and Coombes, J. (2017). A systematic review and meta-analysis of interval training versus moderate-intensity continuous training on body adiposity. Obesity Reviews, [online] 18(8), pp.943-964. Available at: https://www.researchgate.net/publication/317005622_A_systematic_review_and_meta-analysis_of_interval_training_versus_moderate-intensity_continuous_training_on_body_adiposity [Accessed 26 Jun. 2017].

Kid, P. (2010). Vitamins D and K as pleiotropic nutrients: clinical importance to the skeletal and cardiovascular systems and preliminary evidence for synergy. Alternative Medicine Review, [online] 15(3), pp.199-222. Available at: http://www.biomedsearch.com/article/Vitamins-D-K-as-pleiotropic/239916608.html [Accessed 4 Feb. 2017].

Kim, T., Shin, Y., Lee, J., Min, Y. and Yang, H. (2010). Effect of caffeine on the metabolic responses of lipolysis and activated sweat gland density in human during physical activity. Food Science and Biotechnology, [online] 19(4), pp.1077-1081. Available at: http://www.citethisforme.com/cite/journal/autocite [Accessed 7 Mar. 2017].

Kubota, K., Sawada, T., Kita, J., Shimoda, M., Kato, M., Ishizuka, M. and Park, K. (2012). Effect of menatetrenone, a vitamin k2 analog, on recurrence of hepatocellular carcinoma after surgical resection: a prospective randomized controlled trial. Anticancer Research, [online] 32(12), pp.5415-20. Available at: http://ar.iiarjournals.org/content/32/12/5415.full [Accessed 3 Mar. 2017].

Learney, P. (2015). N1 nutritional programming. 1st ed. ACA Publications, p.114.

Lelong, H., Galan, P., Kesse-Guyot, E., Fezeu, L., Hercberg, S. and Blacher, J. (2014). Relationship Between Nutrition and Blood Pressure: A Cross-Sectional Analysis from the NutriNet-Sante Study, a French Web-based Cohort Study. American Journal of Hypertension, [online] 28(3), pp.362-371. Available at: https://academic.oup.com/ajh/article/28/3/362/2743418/Relationship-Between-Nutrition-and-Blood-Pressure [Accessed 28 Feb. 2017].

Levine, J. (2002). Non-exercise activity thermogenesis (NEAT). Best Practice & Research Clinical Endocrinology & Metabolism, [online] 16(4), pp.679-702. Available at: https://www.ncbi.nlm.nih.gov/pubmed/12468415 [Accessed 6 Mar. 2017].

Linde, J., Jeffery, R., French, S., Pronk, N. and Boyle, R. (2005). Self-weighing in weight gain prevention and weight loss trials. Annals of Behavioral Medicine, 30(3), pp.210-216.

Lopresti, A., Maes, M., Maker, G., Hood, S. and Drummond, P. (2014). Curcumin for the treatment of major depression: A randomised, double-blind, placebo controlled study. Journal of Affective Disorders, [online] 167, pp.368-375. Available at: https://www.researchgate.net/publication/269129922_Curcumin_and_major_depression_A_randomised_double-blind_placebo-controlled_trial_investigating_the_potential_of_peripheral_biomarkers_to_predict_treatment_response_and_antidepressant_mechanisms_of_cha [Accessed 12 Jul. 2017].

Martin, W., Armstrong, L. and Rodriguez, N. (2005). Nutrition & Metabolism, [online] 2(1), p.25. Available at: https://nutritionandmetabolism.biomedcentral.com/articles/10.1186/1743-7075-2-25 [Accessed 1 Jul. 2017].

Mcdonald, L. (2008). Do Fat Loss Supplements Work? : Bodyrecomposition. [online] Bodyrecomposition.com. Available at: http://www.bodyrecomposition.com/fat-loss/fat-loss-supplements-2.html [Accessed 3 Mar. 2017].

Mcdonald, L. (2008). The Baseline Diet 2009: Part 1. [online] http://www.bodyrecomposition.com/. Available at: http://www.bodyrecomposition.com/muscle-gain/the-baseline-diet-part-1.html/ [Accessed 23 Dec. 2016].

Mcdonald, L. (2008). The Fundamentals of Fat Loss Diets Part 2 : Bodyrecomposition. [online] Bodyrecomposition.com. Available at: http://www.bodyrecomposition.com/fat-loss/the-fundamentals-of-fat-loss-diets-part-2.html/ [Accessed 9 Nov. 2016].

Mcdonald, L. (2008). The Transition Phase Between Dieting and Gaining - : Bodyrecomposition. [online] Bodyrecomposition.com. Available at: http://www.bodyrecomposition.com/fat-loss/transition-phase-between-dieting-gaining.html/ [Accessed 25 Jan. 2017].

Mcdonald, L. (2008). Warming Up For the Weight Room Part 1 : Bodyrecomposition. [online] Bodyrecomposition.com. Available at: http://www.bodyrecomposition.com/muscle-gain/warming-up-for-the-weight-room-part-1.html/ [Accessed 3 Feb. 2017].

Mente, A., O'Donnell, M., Rangarajan, S., Dagenais, G., Lear, S., McQueen, M., Diaz, R., Avezum, A., Lopez-Jaramillo, P., Lanas, F., Li, W., Lu, Y., Yi, S., Rensheng, L., Iqbal, R., Mony, P., Yusuf, R., Yusoff, K., Szuba, A., Oguz, A., Rosengren, A., Bahonar, A., Yusufali, A., Schutte, A., Chifamba, J., Mann, J., Anand, S., Teo, K. and Yusuf, S. (2016). Associations of urinary sodium excretion with cardiovascular events in individuals with and without hypertension: a pooled analysis of data from four studies. The Lancet, [online] 388(10043), pp.465-475. Available at: http://www.thelancet.com/journals/lancet/article/PIIS0140-6736(16)30467-6/fulltext [Accessed 27 Feb. 2017].

Micha, R., Michas, G. and Mozaffarian, D. (2012). Unprocessed Red and Processed Meats and Risk of Coronary Artery Disease and Type 2 Diabetes â€" An Updated Review of the Evidence. Current Atherosclerosis Reports, [online] 14(6), pp.515-524. Available at: https://www.ncbi.nlm.nih.gov/pmc/articles/PMC3483430/ [Accessed 2 Jan. 2017].

Moyad, M. (2008). Vitamin D: a rapid review. Dermatology Nursing, [online] 28(5), pp.384; quiz 350. Available at: http://www.medscape.com/viewarticle/589256_8 [Accessed 26 Feb. 2017].

Murray, B. (2007). Hydration and Physical Performance. Journal of the American College of Nutrition, [online] 26(sup5), pp.542S-548S. Available at: http://www.tandfonline.com/doi/abs/10.1080/07315724.2007.10719656 [Accessed 4 Feb. 2017].

Nadelen, M. (2016). ACSM | Articles. [online] Acsm.org. Available at: http://www.acsm.org/public-information/articles/2016/10/07/basic-injury-prevention-concepts [Accessed 3 Feb. 2017].

Naimo, M., de Souza, E., Wilson, J., Carpenter, A., Gilchrist, P., Lowery, R., Averbuch, B., White, T. and Joy, J. (2014). High-intensity Interval Training Has Positive Effects on Performance In Ice Hockey Players. International Journal of Sports Medicine, [online] 36(01), pp.61-66. Available at: https://www.researchgate.net/publication/267096096_High-intensity_Interval_Training_Has_Positive_Effects_on_Performance_In_Ice_Hockey_Players [Accessed 6 Feb. 2017].

Naturalproductsinsider.com. (2011). AHA Makes Omega-3 Intake Recommendations. [online] Available at: https://www.naturalproductsinsider.com/news/2011/05/aha-makes-omega-3-intake-recommendations.aspx [Accessed 24 Feb. 2017].

Naude, C., Schoonees, A., Senekal, M., Young, T., Garner, P. and Volmink, J. (2014). Low Carbohydrate versus Isoenergetic Balanced Diets for Reducing Weight and Cardiovascular Risk: A Systematic Review and Meta-Analysis. PLoS ONE, [online] 9(7), p.e100652. Available at: http://journals. plos.org/plosone/article?id=10.1371/journal.pone.0100652 [Accessed 3 Jul. 2017].

Nestle, M. (2017). Why Calories Count: The Problem With Dietary-Intake Studies. [online] The Atlantic. Available at: https://www.theatlantic.com/health/archive/2012/03/ why-calories-count-the-problem-with-dietary-intake-studies/254886/#footnote-1 [Accessed 13 Mar. 2017].

NHS. (2017). The 10,000 steps challenge. [online] Available at: http://www.nhs.uk/livewell/loseweight/pages/ 10000stepschallenge.aspx [Accessed 5 Apr. 2017].
Nhs.uk. (2015). Physical activity guidelines for adults - Live Well - NHS Choices. [online] Available at: http:// www.nhs.uk/Livewell/fitness/Pages/physical-activity-guidelines-for-adults.aspx#moderate [Accessed 5 Feb. 2017].

Nhs.uk. (2015). Why is fibre important? - Health questions - NHS Choices. [online] Available at: http://www.nhs. uk/chq/pages/1141.aspx?categoryid=51 [Accessed 20 Jan. 2017].

Nhs.uk. (2017). Need for eight glasses of water a day questionned - Health News - NHS Choices. [online] Available at: http://www.nhs.uk/news/2011/07July/Pages/eight-glasses-of-water-a-day.aspx [Accessed 19 Aug. 2016].

Norman, A. (2008). From vitamin D to hormone D: fundamentals of the vitamin D endocrine system essential for good health. American Journal of Clinical Nutrition, [online] 88(2), pp.491S-499S. Available at: http://ajcn.nutrition.org/content/88/2/491S.full [Accessed 12 Jul. 2017].

Olsen, O., SjÃ‚haug, M., Van Beekvelt, M. and Mork, P. (2012). The Effect of Warm-Up and Cool-Down Exercise on Delayed Onset Muscle Soreness in the Quadriceps Muscle: a Randomized Controlled Trial. Journal of Human Kinetics, [online] 35(1). Available at: https://www.ncbi.nlm.nih.gov/pubmed/23486850 [Accessed 5 Feb. 2017].

Page, P. (2012). CURRENT CONCEPTS IN MUSCLE STRETCHING FOR EXERCISE AND REHABILITATION. International Journal of Sports Physical Therapy, [online] 7(1), pp.109-119. Available at: https://www.ncbi.nlm.nih.gov/pmc/articles/PMC3273886/ [Accessed 3 Feb. 2017].

Pilz, S., Frisch, S., Koertke, H., Kuhn, J., Dreier, J., Obermayer-Pietsch, B., Wehr, E. and Zittermann, A. (2010). Effect of Vitamin D Supplementation on Testosterone Levels in Men. Hormone and Metabolic Research, [online] 43(03), pp.223-225. Available at: https://www.researchgate.net/profile/Stefan_Pilz/publication/49679775_Effect_of_Vitamin_D_Supplementation_on_Testosterone_Levels_in_Men/links/0c96052f7e9b2ca8d8000000/Effect-of-Vitamin-D-Supplementation-on-Testosterone-Levels-in-Men.pdf [Accessed 28 Feb. 2017].

Poortmans, J. and Dellalieux, O. (2000). Do Regular High Protein Diets Have Potential Health Risks on Kidney Function in Athletes?. International Journal of Sport Nutrition and Exercise Metabolism, [online] 10(1), pp.28-38. Available at: https://www.ncbi.nlm.nih.gov/pubmed/10722779 [Accessed 2 Feb. 2017].

Popkin, B., D'Anci, K. and Rosenberg, I. (2010). Water, hydration, and health. Nutrition Reviews, [online] 68(8), pp.439-458. Available at: https://www.ncbi.nlm.nih.gov/pmc/articles/PMC2908954/ [Accessed 3 Feb. 2017].

Power, C. and HyppÃ¶nen, E. (2007). Hypovitaminosis D in British adults at age 45 y: nationwide cohort study of dietary and lifestyle predictors. American Journal of Clinical Nutrition, [online] 85(3), pp.860-868. Available at: http://ajcn.nutrition.org/content/85/3/860.full [Accessed 27 Feb. 2017].

Ratamess, N., Kraemer, W., Volek, J., Rubin, M., GÃ³mez, A., French, D., Sharman, M., McGuigan, M., Scheett, T., HÃ¤kkinen, K., Newton, R. and Dioguardi, F. (2003). The Effects of Amino Acid Supplementation on Muscular Performance During Resistance Training Overreaching. The Journal of Strength and Conditioning Research, [online] 17(2), p.250. Available at: https://www.researchgate.net/publication/10764203_The_Effects_of_Amino_Acid_Supplementation_on_Muscular_Performance_During_Resistance_Training_Overreaching [Accessed 11 Nov. 2016].

Rey, E., Lago-PeÃ±as, C., CasÃ¡is, L. and Lago-Ballesteros, J. (2012). The Effect of Immediate Post-Training Active and Passive Recovery Interventions on Anaerobic Performance and Lower Limb Flexibility in Professional Soccer Players. Journal of Human Kinetics, [online] 31(-

1). Available at: https://www.ncbi.nlm.nih.gov/pmc/articles/ PMC3588659/ [Accessed 5 Feb. 2017].

Rey, E., Lago-PeÃ±as, C., Lago-Ballesteros, J. and CasÃ¡is, L. (2012). The Effect of Recovery Strategies on Contractile Properties Using Tensiomyography and Perceived Muscle Soreness in Professional Soccer Players. Journal of Strength and Conditioning Research, [online] 26(11), pp.3081-3088. Available at: https://www.researchgate.net/ publication/51973787_The_Effect_of_Recovery_Strategies_ on_Contractile_Properties_Using_Tensiomyography_and_ Perceived_Muscle_Soreness_in_Professional_Soccer_Players [Accessed 5 Feb. 2017].

Schoenfeld, B. (2012). Does Exercise-Induced Muscle Damage Play a Role in Skeletal Muscle Hypertrophy?. Journal of Strength and Conditioning Research, [online] 26(5), pp.1441-1453. Available at: https://www.researchgate.net/ publication/221841567_Does_Exercise-Induced_Muscle_ Damage_Play_a_Role_in_Skeletal_Muscle_Hypertrophy [Accessed 27 Nov. 2016].

Schoenfeld, B. (2017). Â» Are Frequent Meals Beneficial for Body Composition. [online] Lookgreatnaked.com. Available at: http://www.lookgreatnaked.com/blog/are-frequent-meals-beneficial-for-body-composition/ [Accessed 9 Dec. 2016].

Schoenfeld, B. (2017). Â» Does Light Load Training Build Muscle in Experienced Lifters?. [online] Lookgreatnaked.com. Available at: http://www.lookgreatnaked.com/ blog/does-light-load-training-build-muscle-in-experienced-lifters/ [Accessed 25 Apr. 2017].

Schoenfeld, B. (2017). Â» How Many Sets Do You Need to Perform to Maximize Muscle Gains?. [online] Lookgreatnaked.com. Available at: http://www.lookgreatnaked.com/blog/how-many-sets-do-you-need-to-perform-to-maximize-muscle-gains/ [Accessed 10 Jun. 2017].

Schoenfeld, B. and Contreras, B. (2013). Is Postexercise Muscle Soreness a Valid Indicator of Muscular Adaptations?. Strength and Conditioning Journal, [online] 35(5), pp.16-21. Available at: https://www.nsca.com/uploadedfiles/nsca/resources/pdf/certification/quizzes/quiz_pack_articles/october_2013_35.5.pdf [Accessed 28 Nov. 2016].

Schoenfeld, B., Ogborn, D. and Krieger, J. (2016). Dose-response relationship between weekly resistance training volume and increases in muscle mass: A systematic review and meta-analysis. Journal of Sports Sciences, [online] 35(11), pp.1073-1082. Available at: https://www.researchgate.net/publication/305455324_Dose-response_relationship_between_weekly_resistance_training_volume_and_increases_in_muscle_mass_A_systematic_review_and_meta-analysis [Accessed 12 Jul. 2017].

Schoenfeld, B., Ogborn, D. and Krieger, J. (2016). Effects of Resistance Training Frequency on Measures of Muscle Hypertrophy: A Systematic Review and Meta-Analysis. Sports Medicine, [online] 46(11), pp.1689-1697. Available at: https://www.researchgate.net/publication/301578131_Effects_of_Resistance_Training_Frequency_on_Measures_of_Muscle_Hypertrophy_A_Systematic_Review_and_Meta-Analysis [Accessed 28 Apr. 2017].

Schoenfeld, B., Pope, Z., Benik, F., Hester, G., Sellers, J., Nooner, J., Schnaiter, J., Bond-Williams, K., Carter, A., Ross, C., Just, B., Henselmans, M. and Krieger, J. (2016). Longer Interset Rest Periods Enhance Muscle Strength and Hypertrophy in Resistance-Trained Men. Journal of Strength and Conditioning Research, [online] 30(7), pp.1805-1812. Available at: https://www.researchgate.net/profile/Brad_Schoenfeld/publication/284711582_Longer_inter-set_rest_periods_enhance_muscle_strength_and_hypertrophy_in_resistance-trained_men/links/565b792208ae4988a7ba831d/Longer-inter-set-rest-periods-enhance-muscle-strength-and-hypertrophy-in-resistance-trained-men.pdf [Accessed 29 Feb. 2017].

Simopoulos, A. (2002). The importance of the ratio of omega-6/omega-3 essential fatty acids. Biomedicine & Pharmacotherapy, [online] 56(8), pp.365-79. Available at: http://gamalift.com.br/site/artigos/21.pdf [Accessed 26 Feb. 2017].

Siri-Tarino, P., Chiu, S., Bergeron, N. and Krauss, R. (2015). Saturated Fats Versus Polyunsaturated Fats Versus Carbohydrates for Cardiovascular Disease Prevention and Treatment. Annual Review of Nutrition, [online] 35(1), pp.517-543. Available at: https://www.ncbi.nlm.nih.gov/pmc/articles/PMC4744652/ [Accessed 6 Apr. 2017].

Sun, Q. (2012). Red Meat Consumption and Mortality. Archives of Internal Medicine, [online] 172(7), p.555. Available at: https://www.ncbi.nlm.nih.gov/pmc/articles/PMC3712342/ [Accessed 3 Jul. 2017].

Taylor, K., Sheppard, J., Lee, H. and Plummer, N. (2009). Negative effect of static stretching restored when combined with a sport specific warm-up component. Journal of Science and Medicine in Sport, [online] 12(6), pp.657-661. Available at: https://www.researchgate.net/publication/23235253_Negative_effect_of_static_stretching_restored_when_combined_with_a_sport_specific_warm-up_component [Accessed 3 Feb. 2017].

VanWormer, J., Linde, J., Harnack, L., Stovitz, S. and Jeffery, R. (2011). Self-Weighing Frequency Is Associated with Weight Gain Prevention over 2 Years Among Working Adults. International Journal of Behavioral Medicine, [online] 19(3), pp.351-358. Available at: https://www.ncbi.nlm.nih.gov/pmc/articles/PMC3474347/ [Accessed 5 Jan. 2017].

Vitamindcouncil.org. (2017). Vitamin D Council | How do I get the vitamin D my body needs?. [online] Available at: https://www.vitamindcouncil.org/about-vitamin-d/how-do-i-get-the-vitamin-d-my-body-needs/ [Accessed 23 Feb. 2017].

VOLEK, J., DUNCAN, N., MAZZETTI, S., STARON, R., PUTUKIAN, M., G??MEZ, A., PEARSON, D., FINK, W. and KRAEMER, W. (1999). Performance and muscle fiber adaptations to creatine supplementation and heavy resistance training. Medicine & Science in Sports & Exercise, [online] 31(8), pp.1147-1156. Available at: https://www.researchgate.net/publication/12850851_Performance_and_muscle_fiber_adaptations_to_creatine_supplementation_and_heavy_resistance_training [Accessed 2 Feb. 2017].

VOLEK, J., KRAEMER, W., BUSH, J., BOETES, M., INCLEDON, T., CLARK, K. and LYNCH, J. (1997). Creatine Supplementation Enhances Muscular Performance During High-Intensity Resistance Exercise. Journal of the American Dietetic Association, [online] 97(7), pp.765-770. Available at: https://www.researchgate.net/publication/14002113_Creatine_Supplementation_Enhances_Muscular_Performance_During_High-Intensity_Resistance_Exercise [Accessed 8 Feb. 2017].

Volek, J., Kraemer, W., Bush, J., Incledon, T. and Boetes, M. (1997). Testosterone and cortisol in relationship to dietary nutrients and resistance exercise. Journal of Applied Physiology, [online] 82(1), pp.49-54. Available at: http://jap.physiology.org/content/82/1/49 [Accessed 4 Jul. 2017].

Wehr, E., Pilz, S., Boehm, B., MÃƒÂ¤rz, W. and Obermayer-Pietsch, B. (2009). Association of vitamin D status with serum androgen levels in men. Clinical Endocrinology, [online] 73(2), pp.243-8. Available at: http://onlinelibrary.wiley.com/wol1/doi/10.1111/j.1365-2265.2009.03777.x/full [Accessed 28 Feb. 2017].

Westcott, W. (2012). Resistance Training is Medicine. Current Sports Medicine Reports, [online] 11(4), pp.209-216. Available at: http://journals.lww.com/acsm-csmr/Abstract/2012/07000/Resistance_Training_is_Medicine___Effects_of.13.aspx [Accessed 10 Mar. 2017].

Westerterp, K. (2004). Diet induced thermogenesis. Nutrition & Metabolism, [online] 1(1), p.5. Available at: https://nutritionandmetabolism.biomedcentral.com/articles/10.1186/1743-7075-1-5 [Accessed 2 Oct. 2016].

Winett, R. and Carpinelli, R. (2001). Potential Health-Related Benefits of Resistance Training. Preventive Medicine, 33(5), pp.503-513.

Winett, R. and Carpinelli, R. (2001). Potential Health-Related Benefits of Resistance Training. Preventive Medicine, [online] 33(5), pp.503-513. Available at: https://www.ncbi.nlm.nih.gov/pubmed/11676593 [Accessed 26 Jun. 2017].

Wing, R. and Phelan, S. (2005). Long-term weight loss maintenance. The America Journal of Clinical Nutrition, [online] 82(1), pp.222S-225S. Available at: http://ajcn.nutrition.org/content/82/1/222S.long [Accessed 3 Jul. 2017].

Zawadzki, K., Yaspelkis, B. and Ivy, J. (1992). Carbohydrate-protein complex increases the rate of muscle glycogen storage after exercis. Journal of Applied Physiology, [online] 72(5), pp.1854-9. Available at: https://www.researchgate.net/publication/21553526_Carbohydrate-protein_complex_increases_the_rate_of_muscle_glycogen_storage_after_exercise [Accessed 7 May 2017].